MAYO CLINIC

GUIDE TO
PREVENTING & TREATING
Osteoporosis

SECOND EDITION

Bart L. Clarke, M.D.

Medical Editor

Mayo Clinic
Rochester, Minnesota

Mayo Clinic Guide to Treating & Preventing Osteoporosis provides reliable, practical information on understanding and managing this common bone disorder. Much of the information comes directly from the experience of osteoporosis specialists and other health care professionals at Mayo Clinic. This book supplements the advice of your physician, whom you should consult for individual medical problems.

Mayo Clinic Guide to Treating & Preventing Osteoporosis does not endorse any company or product. MAYO, MAYO CLINIC and the Mayo triple-shield logo are marks of Mayo Foundation for Medical Education and Research.

For bulk sales to employers, member groups and health-related companies, contact Mayo Clinic Global Business Solutions, 200 First St. SW, Rochester, MN 55905, or send an email to SpecialSalesMayoBooks@Mayo.edu.

Published by Mayo Clinic

© 2014 Mayo Foundation for Medical Education and Research (MFMER)

Library of Congress Control Number: 2014931451

Second Edition

1 2 3 4 5 6 7 8 9 10

Image credits

The individuals pictured are models, and the photos are used for illustrative purposes only. There's no correlation between the individuals portrayed and the subjects being discussed.

Editorial staff

Medical Editor

Bart L. Clarke, M.D.

Managing Editor

Karen R. Wallevand

Editorial Director

Paula Marlow Limbeck

Product Manager

Christopher C. Frye

Art Director

Richard A. Resnick

Illustration and Photography

Michael A. King

Jodi O'Shaughnessy Olson

James E. Rownd

Research Manager

Deirdre A. Herman

Research Librarian

Erika A. Riggin

Proofreading

Miranda M. Attlesey

Donna L. Hanson

Julie M. Maas

Indexing

Steve Rath

Contributors

Mark E. Bolander, M.D.

Matthew T. Drake, M.D., Ph.D.

Daniel L. Hurley, M.D.

David F. Kallmes, M.D.

Ann E. Kearns, M.D., Ph.D.

Kurt A. Kennel, M.D.

Sundeep Khosla, M.D.

L. Joseph Melton, M.D.

Brian P. Mullan, M.D.

Jennifer K. Nelson, R.D., L.D.

Mehrsheed Sinaki, M.D.

Robert D. Tiegs, M.D.

Robert A. Wermers, M.D.

Administrative Assistant

Beverly J. Steele

Preface

Your life doesn't have to be upended by weakened bones. Osteoporosis was once considered an unfortunate result of growing old. Today — thanks in large part to years of progressive research by investigators at Mayo Clinic and elsewhere — we know that bone loss from osteoporosis can often be avoided or effectively managed. Future generations no longer have to experience the pain and disability once caused by this disease.

This new edition of *Mayo Clinic Guide to Preventing & Treating Osteoporosis* provides updated information on a variety of factors doctors consider in assessing your bone health and your risk of osteoporosis. The book includes a comprehensive, take-charge approach to diagnosing and managing osteoporosis, as well as detailed information and guidance on diet, supplements, exercise, medications and pain control.

You will learn how to reduce your risk of fracture due to falling. You'll also read about the importance of good posture, fitness, and balance and coordination. In addition, there's information on the latest advances in medications and advice on how to evaluate your treatment options.

Mayo Clinic doctors who specialize in osteoporosis have reviewed the chapters to ensure that you receive the most accurate and up-to-date information.

We believe you'll find this book to be a helpful resource for effectively preventing and treating osteoporosis. Use of the strategies described in these pages, together with the support of family and friends and the guidance of your personal physician, can offer you the best opportunity to prevent bone loss and continue to live an active and independent life.

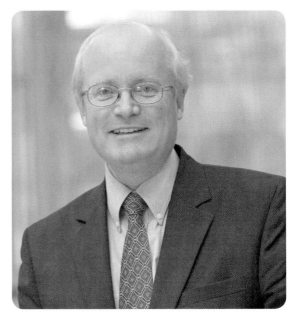

Bart L. Clarke, M.D.
Medical Editor

Table of contents

Preface

Part 1: Understanding Osteoporosis.... 9

Chapter 1   **What is osteoporosis?** 11
     Osteoporosis risks... 12
     Your bone bank 14
     Signs and symptoms 15
     Types 17
     A positive outlook... 20

Chapter 2   **The life cycle of bone** 21
     Bone basics 22
     Bone remodeling... 24
     Hormones and bone formation................................... 26
     Peak bone density.. 28
     Aging and your bones 29
     Maximizing peak bone density 34

Chapter 3   **Fractures and falls** 35
     Fractures.. 36
     Falls... 42
     Avoiding future fractures... 46
     Preventing fractures 48

Chapter 4   **Can you reduce your risk?** 49
     Understanding your risk 50
     Risk factors you can't change 50
     Risk factors you can influence................................... 54
     Risk factors you can change 58
     What's next?...62

Chapter 5 **Screening and diagnosis** **63**

Screening vs. diagnosing 63

What's a bone density test? 65

How testing is done 68

Types of bone densitometers 70

History and physical exam 77

Bone marker tests 78

Making a diagnosis 80

Chapter 6 **Making sense of test results** **81**

What's included 81

Understanding T-scores 85

Understanding Z-scores 87

How are the numbers used? 88

Other risk factors 90

In summary 94

Part 2: Prevention and Treatment 95

Chapter 7 **Developing an action plan** **97**

Strong bones for a lifetime 97

Diet and nutrition 98

Physical activity 107

Medications 108

Healthy behaviors 110

Meeting the challenge 110

Chapter 8 **Eating for healthy bones** **111**

Good nutrition in a nutshell 111

Bone-healthy meals 118

Increasing your calcium intake 124

Calcium supplements 125

Foods to avoid 129

Chapter 9 Staying active **131**

Putting thoughts into action 131

Getting started 133

Exercises for osteoporosis 138

How much exercise? 145

Staying in the game 147

Chapter 10 Taking medications **149**

Bisphosphonates 151

Teriparatide 154

Denosumab 157

Raloxifene 158

Calcitonin 160

Thiazide diuretics 161

Getting the most from treatment 161

Chapter 11 Osteoporosis in men **165**

Bone density in men vs. women 165

How do men get osteoporosis? 167

Screening in men 169

Treatment 171

Take action 176

Chapter 12 Disorders associated with osteoporosis **177**

Endocrine disorders 177

Gastrointestinal disorders 178

Rheumatologic disorders 179

Glucocorticoid-related disease 179

Liver disorders 180

Kidney disorders 181

Transplant surgery 181

Cancer 181

Genetic diseases 184

Kyphosis 184

Immobility 186

Part 3: Living With Osteoporosis 187

Chapter 13 **Healthy living strategies**..**189**
Practice good posture................................. 189
Move safely 191
Boost your emotional health........................ 196
Maintain social connections........................ 202

Chapter 14 **Recovering from a fracture**.....................**205**
Your recovery.. 205
How bone heals 206
Vertebral fractures...................................... 208
Hip fractures 211
Wrist fractures.. 215
Managing chronic pain 219

Chapter 15 **Home safety**..**223**
Staying safe indoors.................................... 224
Assistive devices 227
The importance of attitude 233
Taking control 234

Additional resources................................... 235
Glossary.. 239
Index... 242

Part 1

Understanding osteoporosis

Chapter 1

What is osteoporosis?

You may not think of your bones as being alive, but they are. Every day, your body breaks down old bone and replaces it with new. As you get older, however, the ratio becomes unequal: You lose more bone than you gain. If you lose too much, you can develop the bone disease osteoporosis.

Osteoporosis causes bones to become weak, brittle and prone to fracture. The word *osteoporosis* means "porous bones." It's an apt description of what happens to your skeleton if you have the disease. Due to loss of bone tissue, bones that were once dense and strong may be unable to withstand the stress of even normal activity, such as bending over or twisting to look behind you.

Until recently, osteoporosis was considered a natural part of aging, similar to getting gray hair or developing wrinkles. But there's nothing natural, or healthy, about losing 4 inches of height. And it certainly isn't natural to break a bone from coughing or receiving a hug.

But that's precisely what can happen if you're one of the more than 40 million Americans who have osteoporosis or are at high risk due to reduced bone mass.

The good news is the disease is as preventable and treatable as it is common. The keys to successfully avoiding osteoporosis are building a strong skeleton when you're young and slowing the rate of bone loss as you age. Even if you already have osteoporosis, good nutrition, exercise and medications can slow, or even reverse, its progression. It's never too late to do something about your bone health.

Osteoporosis risks

Each year osteoporosis is responsible for more than 2 million fractures. Typically these fractures occur in the spine, hip or wrist, but they may happen in other bones as well. A compression fracture of the spine causes your vertebrae to collapse and may lead to lost inches of height and a stooped posture. Fractures of the hip can change lives. Only about one-third of those who break a hip return to being as active as they were before the fracture. And nearly one-third go to a nursing home permanently. As if that's not enough, add chronic pain and feelings of anxiety and depression to the mix of problems that osteoporosis can cause.

Osteoporosis is most common among postmenopausal women. If you're a female age 50 or older, you have an eye-opening 50 percent chance of breaking a bone during your remaining lifetime. Statistics indicate your risk of breaking a hip is about the same as your combined risk of developing breast, uterine or ovarian cancer. Although fewer men than women get osteoporosis, men have a higher risk of death after breaking a hip.

Many people have weak bones and don't even know it. That's because

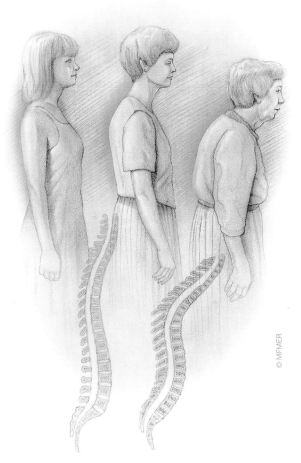

Changes with age Three generations from the same family illustrate how osteoporosis can slowly lead to changes in posture and cause gradual loss of height.

bone loss typically happens over a long period of time and it doesn't hurt. Oftentimes, a broken bone is the first and only indication that a person may have osteoporosis. Unfortunately, by the time a fracture occurs, the disease is often well-established. A bone density test is the best way to predict fracture risk.

Osteoporosis through the ages

Ancient Egyptian mummies with the telltale evidence of hip fractures suggest that osteoporosis has been a problem for humankind through the millennia. But until quite recently, osteoporosis wasn't considered a disease. It was thought to be an inescapable part of aging. Stereotypes from literature, art and even television reinforced this idea. From the old woman who lived in a shoe (of nursery rhyme fame) to Granny on the television series *The Beverly Hillbillies*, older female characters were often portrayed with a tottering walk and stooped over with the so-called dowager's hump.

In the 1830s, a French doctor studying the effects of disease on the human body observed that some people's bones were honeycombed with large holes that greatly weakened the bone structure. He was the first person to describe this condition, which he termed osteoporosis. Unfortunately, the French doctor didn't consider this to be a sign of disease and continued his investigation along different paths.

In the 1940s, Fuller Albright, M.D., of Massachusetts General Hospital, made the connection between the hormone estrogen and osteoporosis. He noticed that many of his patients who had problems with weak bones and fractures were older women past menopause. Dr. Albright believed the sharp drop in estrogen that occurs during menopause was causing the abnormal loss of bone. He correctly identified the condition as postmenopausal osteoporosis.

Still, old notions continued to prevail. Until just the past few decades, women were often told to take calcium and "live with it." But new discoveries have transformed doctors' understanding of the disease. Osteoporosis isn't just an issue for older women. Bone building when you're young and growing is just as important as slowing bone loss as you age.

Your bone bank

Think of your skeleton as a bone bank. Just as your financial health benefits from funds that you put aside and can draw on in times of need, your bone health benefits from a fund of calcium and other minerals that you store in your skeleton. Good bone health depends on keeping your bone bank account amply supplied with minerals that are able to meet all of your body's needs.

Lots of transactions take place in your bone bank account. That's because throughout your life, new bone is constantly being formed and deposited, while old or worn-out bone is

constantly being broken down and withdrawn. By way of this process, your skeleton refurbishes and maintains itself. For adults, the ideal account ledger has as many deposits as it does withdrawals.

Here are some key terms that relate to the bone bank concept. *Bone mass* is the total amount of bone tissue you have in your skeleton. Think of it as the total assets in your account at any time. *Bone density* refers to how tightly that tissue is packed — how mineral-rich your bones are. Envision dollar bills crammed into a safe deposit box. *Bone strength* refers to the ability of bone to withstand stress and is dependent on bone quality, including mass and density. You might compare this to your bank account's ability to handle large daily transactions.

In other words, the more bone you have and the denser it is, the stronger your skeleton — the more plentiful your bone bank account. Strong bones make it less likely that you'll develop osteoporosis or experience fractures.

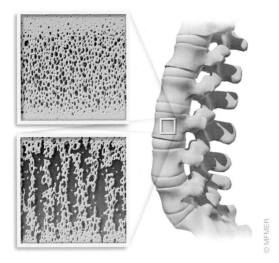

© MFMER

Bone Normal bone is strong and flexible (top left). Osteoporotic bone is more porous, weaker and subject to fracture (bottom left).

Not enough bone in the bank

During your younger years, you're constantly making deposits to your bone

Osteoporosis is not osteoarthritis

Osteoporosis and osteoarthritis are different conditions with very different signs and symptoms, but people sometimes confuse the two. Osteoporosis weakens your bones. Osteoarthritis affects your joints, the locations where bones join to one another. It wears away the cartilage that cushions your bones and keeps them from rubbing against each other. Painful and deformed joints are common signs of osteoarthritis. Osteoporosis often goes unnoticed until a bone is broken.

bank account. But around age 30 things begin to change. Withdrawals from your account begin to exceed your deposits. You gradually start losing bone mass and bone density. This is normal. What's not normal is when withdrawals exceed deposits at such a rate that portions of your skeleton become weak and brittle. Researchers have yet to learn all of the reasons why this occurs. Many factors are likely involved.

Of course, bone loss doesn't mean that you actually lose whole chunks of bone. It's the mineral content of your bones that's depleted. The outer shell of bone becomes thinner, and the interior becomes more porous. This action bankrupts your skeleton of its strength. Under a microscope, a bone affected by osteoporosis looks like a steel bridge with many girders missing. Like a weakened bridge, it may no longer be

able to endure the everyday stresses and strains placed on it.

Your risk of osteoporosis doesn't depend only on your current rate of bone loss. It also depends on how much bone you banked in your account when you were young and growing. This makes the disease equally concerning to a younger person as it is to an older adult.

Signs and symptoms

Osteoporosis is often referred to as a silent thief because the bone loss it causes occurs painlessly over many years. And even in instances when the loss is abnormally rapid, during the

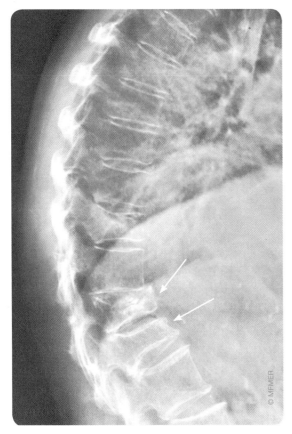

Compression fractures This X-ray image demonstrates how compression fractures of the vertebrae (see arrows) cause abnormal curvature of the spine, resulting in a stooped posture.

early stages you may not experience signs or symptoms.

Then, one day, you break a bone while doing a routine task — maybe you crack a rib while lifting the laundry basket or fracture a vertebra while bending down to tie your shoes. At this point, the disease may already be well-

established and parts of your skeleton may already be quite weak and susceptible to fracture.

Other signs and symptoms may occur if you've experienced a compression fracture of the spine, including:

- Back pain
- Loss of height
- Stooped posture

Remember that back pain, loss of height or stooped posture doesn't mean you have osteoporosis. Only if you've experienced a compression fracture does the disease generally produce back pain. The most common causes of back pain are muscle strain and disk injury. However, because there's the possibility that back pain could stem from an osteoporosis-related fracture, it's important to see a doctor to determine the cause and take appropriate action.

Because, in its early stages, there are no clues that you may be developing osteoporosis, it's important to be aware of factors that put you at increased risk (see Chapter 4). If you're concerned that you may be at increased risk of the disease, have a bone density test before your skeleton becomes weakened. Remember, the best time to act is before you break a bone — not after.

Types

Osteoporosis develops for different reasons. In order to choose the correct course of treatment, your doctor will want to determine the type of osteoporosis you have and what caused it.

In women, osteoporosis most often results from bone loss that occurs after menopause. Often, it's a combination of postmenopausal bone loss combined with age-related bone loss that causes the condition. Most adults reach their peak bone mass in their late 20s or early 30s, and in the years that follow gradually lose mass.

In addition to the effects of age, bone loss may occur as a result of another disease or from the use of certain medications. There are also many secondary forms of osteoporosis, but secondary osteoporosis is less common.

Postmenopausal osteoporosis

Postmenopausal osteoporosis happens during and after menopause as levels of the bone-building hormone estrogen begin to decline. In most women, menopause occurs around age 51. Two to three years before a woman experiences her last menstrual cycle, estrogen levels are already beginning to drop. The reduction continues for another three to four years after the last cycle. During this time, bone loss accelerates because estrogen, which is necessary to maintain your bone health, is no longer present at sufficient levels. Women can lose up to 20 percent of their bone mass during the five to seven years after menopause.

Around age 70, bone loss slows but it doesn't stop. By old age, many women have lost 35 to 50 percent of their bone mass. If you enter menopause with low bone mass, or if you rapidly lose bone after menopause, you're more likely to develop osteoporosis. That's why steps to build and maintain bone mass in your early years are important.

Age-related osteoporosis

All individuals — women and men — lose bone with age. It's normal to lose a small percentage of bone mass each year up to age 80. This happens because as you get older new bone formation slows while bone breakdown stays the same or increases. The internal structure of your bones also weakens, and the outer shell thins. These developments are all a common part of

Secondary causes of osteoporosis in adults

The following medications, conditions and procedures can accelerate bone loss, increasing your risk of osteoporosis:

Medications
- Steroids
- Anticonvulsants
- Excessive thyroid medication
- Certain diuretics, such as loop diuretics
- Certain blood thinners, such as heparin and warfarin
- Certain enzyme inhibitors, such as aromatase inhibitors
- Medications used to treat breast and prostate cancers

Medical conditions
- Endocrine disorders
  - » Sex hormone deficiency (hypogonadism)
  - » Excess parathyroid hormone (hyperparathyroidism)
  - » Cushing's syndrome
  - » Type 1 diabetes
- Stomach, intestinal and liver disorders
  - » Crohn's disease
  - » Celiac disease
  - » Primary biliary cirrhosis
  - » Lactose intolerance
- Rheumatoid arthritis
- Failure to menstruate (amenorrhea)
- Paralysis or prolonged bed rest due to a medical condition

Surgical procedures
- Organ transplant
- Gastric and upper intestinal surgeries

Men get osteoporosis, too

No bones about it, men also get osteoporosis. Beginning in their mid-30s, men start to lose bone mass at a steady rate of about 1 percent a year, and by age 65 they lose bone mass about as fast as women do. From this age on, osteoporosis is as common in men as it is in women.

Because many men think of osteoporosis as a woman's disease, they ignore simple steps to help prevent its development. Approximately 2 million American men have osteoporosis, and another 12 million are at risk of getting it. It's estimated that up to 25 percent of men older than age 50 will break a bone due to osteoporosis. Approximately 80,000 broken hips each year occur in men.

For more information on osteoporosis in men, see Chapter 11.

aging. What's important is the degree of change. It's not normal for you to lose so much bone that you develop osteoporosis.

Osteoporosis is most common in older women because they experience a double whammy. In addition to age-related bone loss, which affects both men and women, older women also are dealing with postmenopausal bone loss. Age-related bone loss may begin before menopause, but its effects often aren't evident until menopause is complete. You may not know that you have age-related bone loss until age 75 or later.

Secondary causes of osteoporosis

Secondary osteoporosis may be related to certain diseases, surgical procedures or medications that accelerate bone loss. Secondary causes are a factor in about 20 to 30 percent of postmenopausal women with osteoporosis and about 50 percent of women approaching menopause (perimenopausal). Among men with osteoporosis, about 50 percent have a secondary cause.

In general, the younger you are when you receive a diagnosis of osteoporosis, the more likely a secondary factor is contributing to the problem. For more information about the causes of secondary osteoporosis, see Chapter 12. The chart on page 18 lists some of the more common factors associated with secondary osteoporosis.

A positive outlook

A bank account is a useful analogy to describe how your skeleton maintains itself and what happens to bones affected by osteoporosis. But this analogy shouldn't be taken too far. Reduced bone density — a low bank account — puts you at increased risk of osteoporosis, but it doesn't mean a bone fracture is a certainty.

Low bone mass and low bone density are good indicators of osteoporosis. However, just as your financial health can't be judged solely by what you've saved in the bank, your bone health isn't based solely on bone density numbers. Your doctor will also take into consideration factors such as your bone structure, age, sex and lifestyle.

Chapter 2

The life cycle of bone

People generally think of bone as being solid and inflexible, even lifeless. To the contrary, your skeleton has an active, if secret, life of its own. Bones are living tissue, involved in a dynamic state of renewal and change.

Within your body, existing bone tissue is continuously being replaced with new bone tissue in what's known as the bone remodeling cycle. At any given moment, millions of bone-removal and bone-building projects are taking place within your skeleton. This process occurs throughout your life, but the balance between how much bone is removed and how much bone is formed varies.

Each stage of your life influences your bone health — starting with fetal growth in the womb and continuing through childhood and adolescence. In your young adult years, your bones grow to their maximum potential in size and density. In the later years of adulthood, the process changes as you begin to lose bone more rapidly than you form it.

Having a basic understanding of the remodeling cycle is important because it can help you comprehend some of the changes that occur to your bone health and bone structure as you age. Keep in mind that the changes vary from person to person because many factors are involved in the remodeling process.

The main point to remember is that positive actions you take now — at any age, but the earlier the better — may help minimize some of the negative effects of age-related change.

Bone basics

Bone's basic structure, its inner framework, is a fibrous meshwork that's composed primarily of the protein collagen. Inlaid within this framework are deposits of minerals such as calcium and phosphorus, with smaller amounts of sodium, magnesium and potassium. These minerals mix with water to form a hard, cement-like substance that makes bone firm and gives it strength.

The outside surface of bone is covered by a thin membrane called the periosteum. This membrane contains blood vessels that supply nutrients to bone, as well as nerves that send pain messages to the brain in case of an injury or disease.

Underneath the membrane covering are three types of tissue that compose bone: cortical bone, trabecular bone and bone marrow.

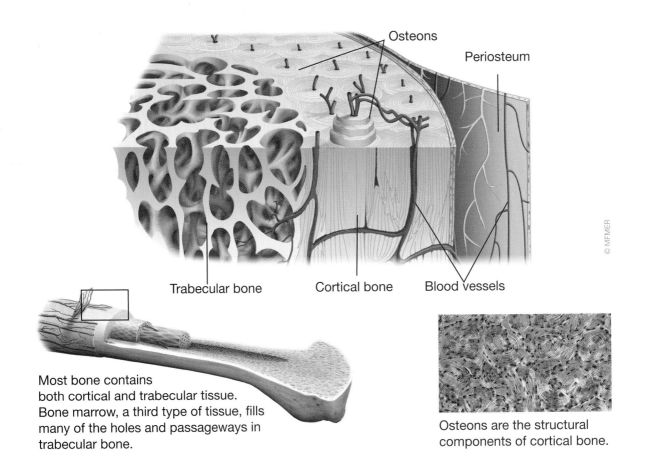

© MFMER

Most bone contains both cortical and trabecular tissue. Bone marrow, a third type of tissue, fills many of the holes and passageways in trabecular bone.

Osteons are the structural components of cortical bone.

Key bone builders

Minerals, like vitamins, are substances that your body needs in certain amounts for normal growth and function. Because your body can't manufacture most minerals and vitamins, you must get them from the foods you eat or, in some cases, from supplements.

Minerals serve many important functions in your body, including the development and maintenance of bone. Bone also serves as a storehouse — or bank — for certain minerals, including calcium, phosphorus and magnesium. When minerals such as these are lacking in your diet, they're extracted from the reserves in your bones. Heavy withdrawals from your bone bank could impair your skeleton's ability to function normally.

Calcium is the most important mineral for bone health. Ninety-nine percent of your body's total calcium is stored in your skeleton. Besides helping keep your bones and teeth strong, calcium is needed for your heart, muscles and nerves to function properly and for your blood to clot normally.

Additional minerals that contribute to bone health and maintenance are phosphate and magnesium and trace amounts of a few others. Most people who eat a balanced diet or who take a standard multivitamin with minerals get sufficient amounts of these minerals.

Cortical bone

Compact (cortical) bone forms the dense outer shell. Its basic components are tightly packed, rod-shaped units called osteons, which look something like long green onions bundled together. Osteons are formed from layers of tissue, much like the layers of an onion. In each layer the collagen fibers face different directions, providing added strength.

Trabecular bone

Cortical bone surrounds a type of spongy tissue called trabecular bone, also referred to as cancellous bone.

Cancellous means "lattice-like." In this type of tissue, millions of tiny interlacing strands, called trabeculae, form a complex latticework structure. Trabeculae are often arranged along the lines of greatest pressure or stress.

This combination of dense cortical tissue with a supple core of trabecular tissue is what makes bones both strong and light. Your skeleton is a tough but somewhat flexible structure that supports your body, protects your brain and other vital organs, and allows you to walk, run, jump, dance and move in many ways.

Most bone contains both cortical and trabecular tissue, but the proportion of each varies from bone to bone. The long bones of the arms, legs and ribs are mostly cortical bone, whereas irregularly shaped bones, such as the pelvis or the vertebrae of the spine, are mostly trabecular bone.

Bone marrow

Bone marrow, the third type of bone tissue, is a soft substance that fills the holes and passageways in the interior of your bones. Bone marrow manufactures your vital oxygen-carrying red blood cells and germ-fighting white blood cells. In long bones, such as the femur in the upper leg, bone marrow fills a canal running through the central shaft.

Bone remodeling

Your skeleton is a never-ending home repair project. Throughout your lifetime, bone tissue is continuously removed and replaced by new bone tissue in a process called bone remodeling (bone turnover). On a regular basis, millions of tiny sections on the surface of your bones are simultaneously under reconstruction — a process unnoticeable to your senses.

Bone remodeling occurs for several important reasons. One is simply to repair damage caused by bone wear and tear. Another is to ensure that enough calcium and other minerals circulate in the bloodstream to carry out the many bodily functions that depend on these minerals. Finally, remodeling is a response to physical activity. Your skeleton adapts to heavier loads and greater stress by forming new bone.

This skeletal regeneration occurs in two basic stages. The initial stage is bone breakdown (resorption), the second is bone formation. Each stage is carried out by a team of specialized bone cells and is regulated by hormones and other substances in the body.

During resorption, cells called osteoclasts become active at locations on the bone surface. These cells attach themselves to the bone and, equipped with special enzymes, begin to break down the surface. As the osteoclasts eat into the bone, proteins and minerals are released and circulated in the bloodstream, sometimes for use in other parts of the body. The activity of the osteoclasts results in microscopic cavities on the surface.

Bone resorption is followed by bone formation, a process carried out by a different group of specialized cells called osteoblasts. The osteoblasts migrate to excavated areas where they begin to fill in the cavities with collagen. Gradually, the meshwork hardens as minerals carried in the bloodstream are redeposited in the collagen. The cycle ends when the collagen is completely mineralized — bone that was removed during resorption is now replaced.

A full cycle of bone remodeling at one site — the excavation of a cavity and the replacement of collagen and minerals in the cavity — takes about three to six months in children and adolescents and six months to a year in adults. In older adults, the process may take up to 18 months.

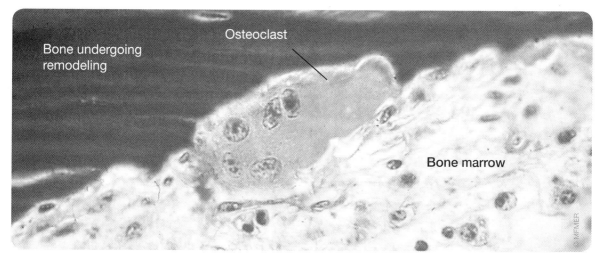

Bone resorption This microphotograph shows a specialized bone cell, called an osteoclast, breaking down the bone surface during resorption.

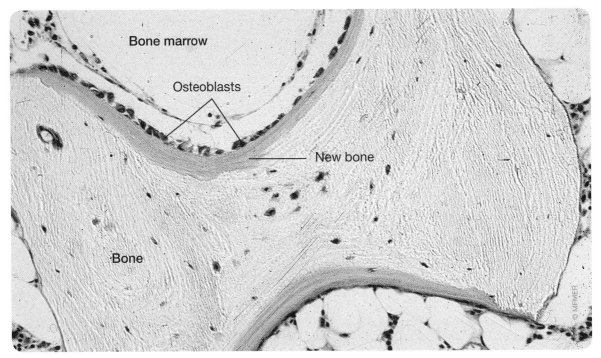

Bone formation This microphotograph of bone formation shows a line of specialized bone cells, called osteoblasts, at work forming new bone.

As tends to be true with most remodeling projects, the demolition phase generally goes faster than the reconstruction phase. Therefore, to maintain your skeleton at any given moment, fewer sections are being broken down than are being rebuilt.

For individuals in their 30s, about 1 percent of the skeleton is undergoing bone breakdown while about 4 percent is undergoing bone formation. At this pace, your skeleton undergoes complete regeneration every 10 years.

Hormones and bone formation

The activities of osteoclasts and osteoblasts in the bone remodeling cycle are controlled by hormones and other substances that allow bone cells to communicate with one another. Hormones also affect how much calcium is extracted from your food and how much calcium is eliminated from your body.

The word *hormone* means "to excite" or "to spur on." Hormones are chemical messengers that target specific parts of the body to help regulate many processes and functions. Hormones are part of the endocrine system, which is a system of specialized glands. The glands produce and secrete hormones into the bloodstream as they're needed. Because the endocrine system is involved in bone remodeling, endocrinologists are among the specialists who treat osteoporosis.

The main hormone involved in bone remodeling is parathyroid hormone (PTH), which is produced by four small glands located at the base of your neck. When the level of calcium in your bloodstream drops, the parathyroid glands secrete PTH. The hormone stimulates osteoclasts to break down bone and release more calcium. Under special conditions, PTH can also stimulate bone formation.

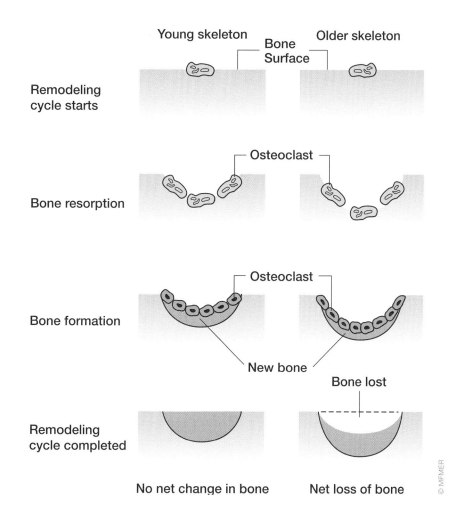

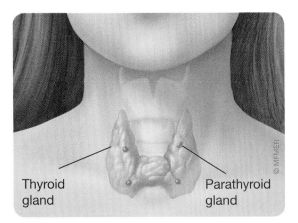

Thyroid gland

Parathyroid gland

© MFMER

Parathyroid glands There are four parathyroid glands (indicated by the gray dots), which lie behind the thyroid gland. The parathyroid glands produce parathyroid hormone, which is vital to your bone health.

The hormone PTH activates vitamin D, which is necessary to increase the amount of calcium absorbed in the gastrointestinal tract and to maintain the calcium balance in the bloodstream. Besides PTH, other substances help regulate bone remodeling. These include calcitonin — a hormone produced by the thyroid gland — and the sex hormones estrogen and testosterone.

You maintain bone strength when the amount of bone that's removed during resorption is fully replaced by new bone. Many factors figure into this equation, including age, hormones, diet and exercise. There's great variation from one person to another and from one stage of life to another. Throughout childhood, adolescence and young adulthood — the prime years of physical growth — more bone is formed than is removed, creating a positive mineral balance in your bone bank. Later in life, changes in your body shift the cycle from surplus bone formation or equilibrium to bone loss.

Peak bone density

When you're young, your skeleton grows to keep pace with other developments of childhood, adolescence and young adulthood. Consequently, during this time your bones grow larger, denser and stronger, and your bone mass increases. At the end of the adolescent growth spurt, young people usually have obtained up to 60 percent of their total adult bone mass. By age 18, longitudinal growth (height) is nearly complete.

Your bone mass typically reaches its maximum in your late 20s to early 30s. This is known as peak bone density — the highest amount of bone mass that you're able to attain as a result of normal growth. At this point, your bones are as fully developed as they'll ever be.

Peak bone density varies from one person to another. It's influenced by:

- **Heredity.** Genetic factors account for about three-fourths of the variation in peak bone density among groups of individuals.
- **Sex.** Peak bone density is generally higher in men than it is in women because men's bones are larger.
- **Race.** Whites and people of Asian descent generally have a lower bone density than do blacks, Hispanics and American Indians.
- **Diet.** People with adequate calcium and vitamin D in their diets generally reach a higher peak bone mass than do individuals who don't get enough calcium and vitamin D.
- **Physical activity.** Exercise and activity are positive skeletal influences because your bones respond to physical activity by becoming denser and stronger.
- **Hormone production.** Estrogen, testosterone and other hormones contribute to bone formation and the maintenance of your skeleton.
- **Medical conditions.** Some chronic medical disorders and certain severe illnesses may affect bone and reduce bone density.
- **Lifestyle.** Smoking and alcohol abuse may have an adverse effect on bone density.

The higher your peak bone density, the better protected you'll be from osteoporosis, and the less likely you'll be to experience a fracture. That's because it takes longer for the effects of aging or illness to weaken strong bones to the point where they easily fracture.

If you're young, a great way to protect yourself from osteoporosis is to develop habits and behaviors that build bone mass. If you're past the age of achieving peak bone mass, don't despair. Many of the same habits and behaviors are effective in preventing or slowing bone loss.

Aging and your bones

Bone remodeling continues after you reach peak bone density, but the balance between formation and resorption shifts. With age, the rate of bone breakdown begins to overtake that of bone formation, and the number of resorption sites increases.

The bottom line is that because your bone density is decreased, the bones that form your skeleton become more porous and brittle.

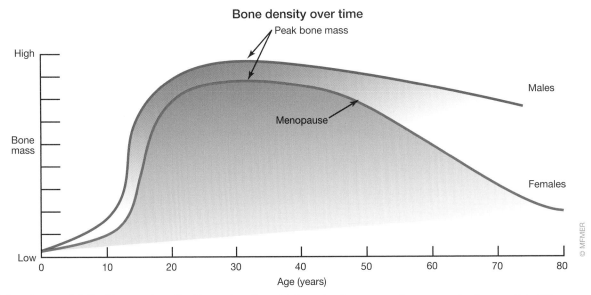

Bone density over time

High

Bone mass

Low

0   10   20   30   40   50   60   70   80

Age (years)

Peak bone mass

Menopause

Males

Females

© MFMER

The rise and fall of bone density Bone density, which varies by sex and race, peaks in your late 20s to early 30s and then slowly declines with age. Women experience a significant decline in bone density after menopause. In general, the higher your peak bone density, the lower your risk of having fractures due to osteoporosis later in life.

The transition from bone gain to bone loss is slow. It's also universal, affecting both men and women, although at different stages in life. In a decade, you'll experience about 3 to 5 percent loss of bone. This change primarily affects trabecular bone, which is less dense than is cortical bone.

The reasons behind the changes to the bone cycle are complex and not completely understood. As you get older, osteoblasts — the bone-forming cells — become less active and new bone is formed more slowly. Changes in your body's ability to absorb calcium along with a decrease in your activity level and lower levels of certain hormones also play a role.

As people age, their intestines gradually absorb less calcium from the foods they eat, so less of the mineral reaches the bloodstream. The kidneys also appear to lose some of their ability to conserve calcium, and as a result more calcium is lost in urine.

Some people also find that as they get older they're less tolerant of the sugar (lactose) in calcium-containing products, such as milk or yogurt.

Are you shrinking?

You probably reached your full adult height by about age 18 — and assumed you'd always remain that tall. Instead, as you enter middle age and beyond, you may find yourself getting shorter. How can that happen?

From day to day, no matter what your age, the disks that cushion and separate the vertebrae in your spine are being compressed during your waking hours. At night, while you rest, the disks have a chance to rehydrate and expand. You may actually be slightly taller in the morning than you are in the evening.

Over time, however, the disks within your vertebrae naturally shrink, causing everyone to lose a little height. This loss may range from about 1 to 3 inches. Osteoporosis can cause the vertebrae in your spine to compress or even collapse, leading to a greater loss of height than normal. Another cause of stooped posture is the weakening of your upper back muscles.

If you feel that you're "shrinking," talk to your doctor. He or she may suggest you be screened for osteoporosis.

Osteoporotic
bone

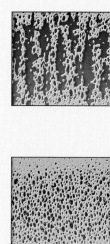

Normal bone

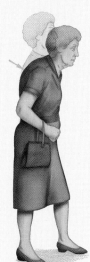

One of the possible long-term effects of osteoporosis is a series of compression fractures that can produce a stooped posture and the appearance of a hump on the upper back.

© MFMER

Because of this, they don't eat as many dairy products, resulting in less calcium. Some people also feel that dairy products contribute to constipation.

Vitamin D production also may drop off as you age. The major source of vitamin D is sunlight, and many adults spend less time in the sun as they get older. With age your skin also becomes less efficient at synthesizing vitamin D from the sun's rays.

In addition, if you're consuming fewer dairy products, it's likely that you're also getting less vitamin D from your diet. With less of the vitamin to help with calcium absorption, much of the calcium you consume may not be making it to your bloodstream.

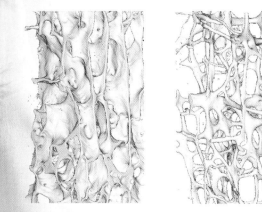

© MFMER

Bone becomes more brittle Three-dimensional images of trabecular bone from a vertebra that compares healthy bone (left) with bone that has been weakened by osteoporosis (right).

Going through menopause

Menopause, which normally starts around age 51, occurs when a woman's ovaries begin making less estrogen. Menstrual periods become irregular and then stop altogether. This transition may take less than a year or more than two years to complete. Declining levels of estrogen and other reproductive hormones are responsible for many of the physical and emotional changes that women may experience during this time.

Estrogen plays a variety of roles in your body. It signals your reproductive organs to mature, and it stimulates your sex drive. Estrogen also has a protective effect on bone, promoting greater density and helping regulate bone remodeling. When your ovaries produce less estrogen, bones lose the hormone's protective effect, and the rate of bone loss increases. This bone loss is irreversible, putting postmenopausal women at high risk of osteoporosis.

The estrogen factor

After menopause bone loss speeds up dramatically in women. This acceleration is primarily due to decreasing levels of the hormone estrogen. A woman may lose as much as 20 percent of her bone mass in the five to seven years after menopause.

Men produce small amounts of estrogen, in addition to testosterone. Although men don't experience comparable bone loss at midlife, lower estrogen levels do affect men's bone density as well.

Around age 70 or 75, the accelerated pace at which women lose bone begins to slow, but it doesn't stop entirely. Bone loss continues with age, but at a slower rate. Ultimately, a woman may lose 35 to 50 percent of her peak bone mass. Men, in comparison, may lose 20 to 30 percent.

It's not surprising then, that women are more likely to develop osteoporosis than are men, and more likely to experience a bone fracture. A woman's peak bone mass is generally lower to begin with, and women experience accelerated loss of bone after menopause. Men generally have larger skeletons and more bone mass, so bone loss caused by aging is less detrimental.

Maximizing peak bone density

Much about the bone remodeling cycle is determined by your genes, and a certain amount of bone loss can be expected as you age. The amount of calcium and other minerals deposited in your bone bank during peak bone formation is critical. A high peak bone mass can counteract or cushion the impact of bone loss in your later years and may reduce your risk of fracture.

There are many things you can do to influence the bone cycle:

- Eat a balanced diet that contains adequate calories, vitamins and minerals, especially calcium and vitamin D.
- Get regular exercise because physical activity contributes to higher bone mass.
- Limit alcohol and don't smoke. Alcohol may interfere with calcium absorption and tobacco is known to contribute to weak bones.

- For teenage females just starting to menstruate, avoid excessive dieting and other behaviors that can interfere with the timing of menstrual periods.

Remember that it's never too late to begin making bone-saving lifestyle changes. Even if you're past the age of peak bone mass, what you eat and drink and how much you exercise can still help keep your bones strong and healthy. For more information on diet and exercise, see Chapters 8 and 9.

Chapter 3

Fractures and falls

Afracture occurs when a bone can't withstand the physical force that's exerted on it. A fracture is often the result of a fall, a sharp blow or another type of traumatic impact. Many people sustain one or more fractures during their lifetime.

When you were a child, a broken bone may have been painful, but the incident — such as falling out of a tree and breaking your arm — likely made for a good story later on. Plus, you got to wear a cool-looking cast. And you may have thought it was really great that everyone signed the cast and drew funny faces on it.

For older adults, however, breaking a bone can be a serious event, resulting in complications that may severely reduce their independence or even prove fatal.

For this reason, preventing fractures and falls in older adults is a major focus of the health care profession.

A bone fracture is the clearest — and often only — indication of osteoporosis. Each year, osteoporosis leads to more than 2 million fractures in the United States. A little more than 25 percent are spinal fractures, while approximately 20 percent are wrist fractures and 15 percent are hip fractures.

When your bone density is reduced, your bones are weakened and they're less able to withstand the pressures and strains of everyday activities. Many times, a bone fracture isn't the result of a traumatic event but rather an event that you would normally consider routine, such as lifting a bag of groceries or a basket of laundry.

Fractures

As discussed in Chapter 2, the balance in the bone remodeling cycle between bone breakdown (resorption) and bone formation changes with age. Break-down starts to occur at a faster rate than does formation. As a result, bone density decreases and open spaces within the bone structure widen. This contributes to a loss of bone mass and much lighter, weaker bones.

Fractures may occur in any bone in your body, but the most common fractures from osteoporosis are of the vertebrae and the hip — bones that directly support your weight. Wrist fractures also are common. Fractures may also occur in the pelvis and the long bones, such as the thighbone and the humerus.

And you don't always have to experience a fall or an injury for a fracture to occur. The vertebrae of your spine can weaken from daily wear and tear, leading to compression fractures. Hip and wrist fractures, however, usually result from a fall. With proper rehabilitation, most people do well following surgical treatment for hip fractures. But some fractures may lead to disability or death. This is usually due to a coexisting condition or disease.

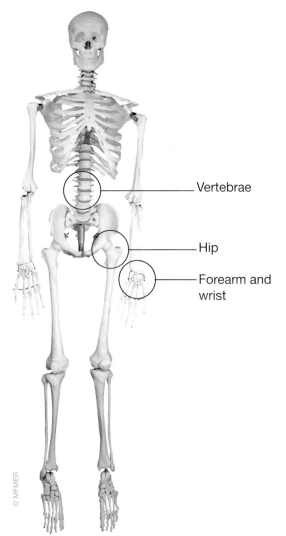

Vertebrae

Hip

Forearm and wrist

© MFMER

Common fracture sites Fractures due to osteoporosis are most likely to occur in the highlighted locations.

Spinal fractures

Your vertebrae support your body, allow you to stand upright and protect the nerves of your spinal cord.

Compression fractures caused by osteoporosis occur when your vertebrae lose bone density to the point of collapse. The front part of the vertebral body literally caves in. These types of fractures usually happen in the lower (lumbar) and middle (thoracic) parts of the spine.

Most compression fractures occur as a result of a routine activity, such as bending over, coughing, sneezing or lifting a small object. Unlike hip fractures, most vertebral fractures aren't related to a fall. If the bone density within your vertebrae is low, just one instance of an activity such as coughing or sneezing is enough to cause a fracture.

A compression fracture often goes undetected. Only about one-third of people with a spinal fracture seek medical attention for the fracture. Sometimes a vertebral fracture can be painful. The pain may start out as a constant nagging or come on suddenly. You may also have some tenderness around the area of the damaged vertebra.

Signs of multiple compression fractures include loss of height and a forward curvature of the spine, an appearance of slouching or slumping over. In a condition known as kyphosis, the curvature of the spine is so exaggerated that it makes you appear as if you have a hump on your back.

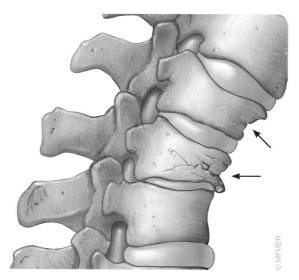

Fractured vertebrae Osteoporosis may cause vertebrae to fracture and compress (see arrows) as a result of weakness in the bone structure.

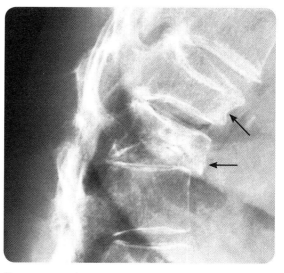

Compressed vertebrae An X-ray image of collapsed vertebrae (see arrows) demonstrates how the spine can develop an abnormal curvature.

Your flexible spine

Your spine is made up of interlocking bones called vertebrae, which are stacked one on top of another in a column. Each vertebra consists of the barrel-shaped vertebral body and bony projections that form the vertebral arch, which protects the spinal cord. Separating the vertebrae are cartilage disks that act as shock absorbers, absorbing the bumps and jolts of everyday life. Your vertebrae form four curves that enhance your body's flexibility and balance.

From top to bottom, the spine's vertebrae become larger and thicker. The seven cervical vertebrae at the top are small and delicate. They support your head. The 12 thoracic vertebrae support your arms and trunk, and the five lumbar vertebrae — the biggest and strongest — support the weight of most of your body and give you a stable center of gravity. Below the lumbar vertebrae, five smaller vertebrae are fused together to form the sacrum.

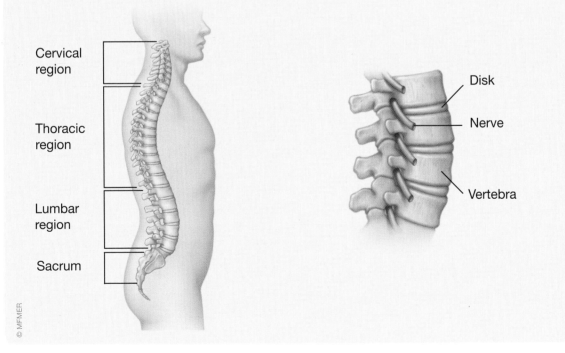

Cervical region

Thoracic region

Lumbar region

Sacrum

Disk

Nerve

Vertebra

© MFMER

If a vertebral fracture isn't causing pain, treatment for the fracture itself may not be necessary. However, it's very important the underlying osteoporosis be treated to prevent future fractures.

Hip fractures

A hip fracture is the most serious outcome of osteoporosis. It's most often the result of a fall, especially when falling sideways or backward. Every year more than 250,000 Americans are hospitalized for a hip fracture. Doctors expect that number to grow as the U.S. population ages.

Because older women lose bone density at a faster rate than do older men, they're two to three times as likely to experience a hip fracture. Men, however, have a higher death rate in the year following a hip fracture, mostly due to coexisting diseases and complications of fracturing. Approximately 1 in 5 individuals who experience a hip fracture die within a year of the incident.

The vast majority of all hip fractures occur at one of two locations along the femur, the long bone that extends from your pelvis to your knee (see page 40):

- **The femoral neck.** This is a thin section of the upper femur located just below its rounded end that fits into the ball-and-socket joint of your hip.
- **The intertrochanteric region.** This is the part of your upper femur immediately below the femoral neck.

Often your doctor can determine that you have a hip fracture based on your signs and symptoms and by observing the abnormal position of your hip and leg. An X-ray can confirm that a bone is broken and reveal exactly which part of the hip is fractured.

Although a hip fracture is usually treatable, complications from the fracture, such as a blood clot or pneumonia, can be life-threatening, particularly for older adults with other serious medical conditions such as heart disease or diabetes.

If you experience a hip fracture and are immobile for a long period, you risk developing blood clots. It's possible for a blood clot to become lodged in a blood vessel in the lung, blocking blood flow to the lung tissue and causing an obstruction (embolism). This condition can be fatal if not treated promptly. Other risks of immobility due to hip fracture include bedsores and urinary tract infection.

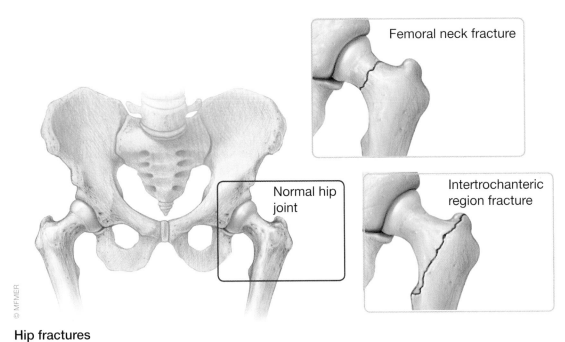

© MFMER

Hip fractures

Most hip fractures occur in one of two locations: the femoral neck or the intertrochanteric region.

Many older adults — including those older than age 80 — do recover from a hip fracture, although the recuperation period can take up to a year, and recovery isn't always complete.

During recovery many people need assistance getting around their homes and doing daily tasks, such as bathing, dressing and cooking. A considerable number of individuals who break a hip enter a long-term care facility while recuperating because they need assistance that's unavailable at home. Generally, the better your health and mobility before the fracture, the better your chances are for a complete recovery.

Wrist fractures

When you feel yourself falling, your natural instinct is to extend your arms to help break the impact of the fall. If the force of the fall is greater than the strength of your wrist bones, the result is often a wrist fracture.

The two main bones of your forearm are the radius and the ulna. The most common location for a wrist fracture among people with osteoporosis is at the end of the radius, just below the wrist. This type of break is called a Colles' fracture. Sometimes both the radius and the ulna are broken by a fall.

Common signs and symptoms of a Colles' fracture include swelling, tenderness or pain in the wrist area. It's also likely that you'll find it difficult to pick up or hold anything of moderate weight. Sometimes the wrist is deformed, inclined at an angle toward the palm of your hand. An X-ray can help your doctor determine the exact location and extent of the injury.

Many people recover from a Colles' fracture without problems, but older adults are at a higher risk of complications and don't always regain full mobility of the wrist joint.

Possible complications may include chronic pain resulting from ligament or joint damage or from arthritis in the wrist. Carpal tunnel syndrome may be another long-term complication if the median nerve, which runs between the radius and the ulna, has been injured and becomes inflamed.

Kids and fractures

A broken bone is often a normal part of an active childhood. About 1 in 3 children experiences a bone fracture. But a recent Mayo Clinic study found certain types of fractures may have implications for a child's long-term bone health.

Researchers found that children who experienced forearm fractures as a result of mild trauma often had lower bone strength than did children whose fractures occurred from moderate or severe trauma.

The researchers say fractures resulting from mild trauma may suggest an underlying skeletal deficit that could increase the risk of osteoporosis later in life. Interventions at a young age to optimize bone strength — including a healthy diet and plenty of weight-bearing exercise — may help reduce this risk.

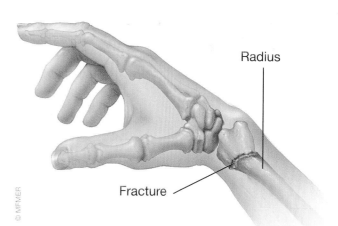

Common wrist fracture A Colles' fracture occurs at the end of the radius, just below the wrist. If you have a wrist fracture, you may feel a sharp pain in your wrist, especially when you try to rotate your hand in a circular motion.

Falls

Falling is one of the major reasons why older adults break bones. Slips and falls can happen to anyone for any reason — a loose carpet, a slick surface, an unexpected change in the pathway, or dizziness caused by a disorder or medication. As you age, a fall becomes more common because you may be less able to effectively react to the situation.

Various changes associated with aging — such as problems with balance, loss of muscle mass and poor vision — can contribute to slower reaction times. Older adults also lose some of their bone strength and fatty cushioning, particularly around the pelvis, which help to break falls.

About a third of people older than age 65 fall at least one time each year. When injury occurs, about one-third of the injuries are fractures. Here's a closer look at some of the main risk factors for falling, including some that you can influence or control.

Problems with balance

As you age, your sense of balance tends to decline and your reaction time slows, increasing the likelihood of falling.

Under normal circumstances, balance is controlled by the signals sent to your brain from three sensory systems in your body:

- **Inner ear.** The slightest movement of your head activates sensors in your inner ear. These sensors send electrical signals to the brain, which is constantly monitoring the position of your head relative to the ground.
- **Eyes.** Visual signals help you determine where your body is within the environment.
- **Sensory nerves.** Nerves in your skin, muscles and joints send messages to your brain about the movement of your body.

Good balance depends on at least two of these systems working well. For instance, closing your eyes while washing your hair in the shower doesn't mean you'll lose your balance — signals from your inner ear and sensory nerves help keep you upright.

If your central nervous system is slow to process these signals, if the messages are contradictory or if your sensory systems aren't functioning properly, your balance may suffer. This may make it harder for you to avoid something in your path or adjust

The mechanics of a fracture

Some osteoporosis research has used engineering principles to calculate the risk of fracture. The amount of force applied to the hip or the spine by certain activities or actions is compared with the maximum amount of pressure these bones can bear — similar to calculating the tonnage a bridge can bear. Researchers were able to identify several activities and actions that involve a high risk of fracture.

One of the most significant risk factors for a hip fracture is falling sideways — either while walking or standing. The impact often exceeds the capacity of an average older adult's hip to sustain the fall, resulting in a fracture. Other factors also influence the risk of fracture. For example, absorbing some of the energy of the fall with your leg muscles or using an outstretched hand to break the fall can reduce the impact on your hip. Skin and fat around the area of impact or padded clothing also can reduce damage caused by the fall.

The risk of a compression fracture in the spine also has been measured. By bending over at a 30-degree angle and lifting a weight of approximately 17 pounds — the equivalent of lifting a small child or a bag of groceries — you more than double your risk of a compression fracture if your bone density is low.

Fracturing your hip The impact when you fall sideways often results in a hip fracture.

to a sudden change in the ground surface, leading to a fall. Some older adults have increased body sway while standing still, which also may increase their risk of falling.

Vision problems

Much like the tissue of your ligaments and tendons, the tissue of the lenses of your eyes become less elastic with age. This reduced elasticity makes it more difficult to focus an image on your retina and to see close objects clearly. Vision problems or changes in your depth perception make it easier for you to trip or stumble off a step.

Many age-related vision problems can be corrected with the right glasses, and older adults may find it necessary to wear bifocals or trifocals to improve vision. However, shifting your eyes between different focal powers in a lens can momentarily disorient you, affecting your balance. This can sometimes lead to a fall. Focusing straight ahead and lowering your head can help avoid this.

Eye conditions such as cataracts, glaucoma and macular degeneration also can affect your perception or make it difficult to see obstacles.

Poor bone quality

There is a direct correlation between the quality of your bones and your risk of fracture. The better your bone quality, the less your risk of fracture. The poorer your bone quality, the greater your risk.

What constitutes bone quality? Your bone quality is generally determined by the rate of bone turnover and the microarchitecture of your bones. These features can be measured to some degree by way of bone marker tests.

Typically, the faster old bone is resorbed and new bone is formed, the weaker the bone. Bones that are less mineral rich and more porous also are more likely to fracture than bones that are more mineral rich and more tightly packed. Bone marker tests are discussed in Chapter 5.

Muscle weakness

As you get older, your muscles tend to lose some of their bulk and they begin to weaken. With time, your ligaments and tendons — the body's connective tissues — also lose their elasticity, which can cause your muscles and joints to stiffen. Lack of physi-cal activity also can decrease muscle mass and strength.

When combined with changes in balance brought on by aging, muscle weakness can turn a stumble into a fall. When your brain receives a signal that you've lost your balance, it immediately triggers your muscles to try and compensate. But if your reaction is slowed and your muscles are weak, your body may be unable to maintain its upright position.

Chronic medical conditions

Chronic medical conditions, which tend to become more common with age, may increase your chances of falling. Conditions that affect your nervous system, such as stroke, Parkinson's disease and multiple sclerosis, may affect your balance and coordination. Disorders affecting your feet and legs, such as arthritis and peripheral nerve damage, may disrupt your ability to walk.

Other chronic conditions that make it difficult to get around — such as emphysema, congestive heart failure or severe obesity — can lead to physical inactivity and loss of muscle strength and balance.

People with decreased mental alertness, such as that caused by dementia or depression, are at increased risk of falling. In addition, flu, low blood pressure or dehydration can cause dizziness.

Reaction to medications

Some drugs can affect your balance and cause dizziness. These include certain blood pressure medications, sedatives, tranquilizers, antidepressants, cold and allergy medications (antihistamines), pain relievers, and sleep medications. Other side effects from medications may include muscle weakness, shakiness and blurred vision, any of which can lead to a fall.

Some of these medications, particularly blood pressure medications, tranquilizers and antidepressants, may cause a sudden drop in blood pressure if you stand up quickly, leading to lightheadedness or fainting. Getting up slowly from a sitting or lying position helps prevent this sudden drop in blood pressure.

Always ask your doctor about the side effects of medications you're taking and how you might reduce these side effects. Your doctor may be able to prescribe a different drug.

Environmental hazards

Factors that aren't related to your physical health also can cause a tumble. Although you may think that your home is a safe place to be, many falls and resulting fractures occur at home.

Some potential hazards within the house include loose rugs, cluttered floors, poor lighting, exposed electrical or telephone cords, and stairs with no handrails. Walking around the house in slippery socks or standing on something other than a sturdy step stool when reaching for an object also can spell trouble.

Any of these hazards could cause you to fall, often onto furniture, increasing your chance of a fracture. For information on making your home safer, see Chapter 15, which also offers tips on preventing falls.

Avoiding future fractures

Most doctors regard fractures caused by routine activities — those that normally wouldn't be traumatic enough to break a bone — as strong evidence of osteoporosis. This kind of fracture is known as a low-trauma fracture.

Compression fractures of the spine, which can occur simply from bending too far forward, all too frequently go unnoticed until osteoporosis is well-developed.

Having a low-trauma fracture increases your risk of future fractures. Statistics show that once you've experienced one fracture, your chances of another fracture are even greater. Studies indicate that a prior fracture is associated with an 86 percent increased risk of another fracture.

According to guidelines published by the American Association of Clinical Endocrinologists, the two most important risk factors for osteoporosis-related fractures are low bone density and a previous low-trauma fracture.

If you fracture a bone, is there something you can do to reduce your chances of a future fracture? The answer is yes. First, see a doctor and consider having a bone density test if you haven't already done so.

According to the World Health Organization, any woman experiencing a wrist fracture after menopause has sufficient cause to evaluate her bone density for osteoporosis. The National Osteoporosis Foundation recommends bone density testing for all postmenopausal women following a fracture. Some doctors may perform a less expensive screening test first and then schedule a more complete bone density test if the screening exam indicates additional testing is warranted.

Other testing may also be done. In addition to checking your hormone levels, your doctor may recommend other tests, including blood tests to check calcium and phosphate levels, thyroid function, and liver function. Urine tests also may be performed.

If your bone density is low, you want to find out the cause — whether it's osteoporosis or some other condition that's leaching minerals from your bones. Once the cause is known, measures can be taken to increase bone density and help strengthen your bones and muscles. With proper treatment your risk of a second fracture may eventually return to normal.

Regardless of the results, don't forget that measuring your bone density is important because it provides a benchmark for determining future changes in your bone health.

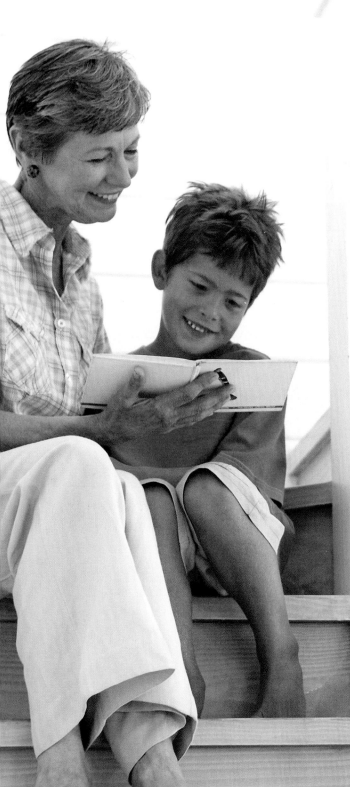

Preventing fractures

Bone fractures can be life-changing events, particularly for older adults. Even a single fracture can put you at greater risk of more fractures, potentially creating a downward spiral in your health.

If you have osteoporosis but are lucky enough to never experience a fracture, your condition may not cause you any serious health problems. That's why it's important to avoid breaking a bone. You can do this by treating your condition, taking steps to prevent falls, and practicing safe movements and activities.

If you've already experienced a fracture, many of the same steps still apply — they can help you prevent future fractures.

The chapters that follow provide more information on protecting your bones. Remember, it's much easier and less expensive to prevent a fracture than it is to treat one.

Chapter 4

Can you reduce your risk?

No one can say for sure whether you'll develop osteoporosis. The disease is too complex for that. But doctors do know what makes some people more likely than others to get it. So it's important to be aware of the risk factors for osteoporosis and understand what you can do to reduce some of them.

If you already have osteoporosis, bone loss has already weakened your skeleton. But if you never experience a fracture, you'll avoid the most serious consequence of the disease. Pain is normally not associated with osteoporosis unless you have a fracture. Even individuals with very low bone density can continue to lead active, independent lives and participate in activities they enjoy, as long as they don't break a bone.

Generally speaking, your risk of osteoporosis and a bone fracture depends on your bone health — the size and strength of your bones and the condition of your bone tissue. Bone health is a result of how well your skeleton developed during childhood and early adulthood and how much bone was present at the time you reached peak bone mass, which usually occurs by your late 20s to early 30s. Bone health is also affected by how rapidly you lose bone mass as you get older.

Many unique factors about you put an individual stamp on your bone health. Those factors include your family history and the genes you inherited, as well as hormones, your diet, the amount of exercise you get, lifestyle behaviors, and your overall state of health.

Factors that reduce your peak bone mass or accelerate bone loss increase your susceptibility to osteoporosis. They're called risk factors. However, by taking precautions, having realistic expectations of what you can or can't do, and doing all that you can to build or maintain bone mass, you can lower your risk of osteoporosis or a fracture.

Understanding your risk

If you were to characterize the person most likely to get osteoporosis, you might describe a tall, thin, white woman past menopause who smokes, abuses alcohol, eats poorly, doesn't exercise and takes medications such as corticosteroids. In addition, her mother would have experienced a stooped posture from multiple compression fractures of the spine.

But keep in mind, even if you share some of these characteristics, you're not necessarily destined to get osteoporosis. And if you do develop the disease, you're not necessarily going to break a bone. Conversely, some people with no known risk factors can develop osteoporosis and break a hip.

If some of the following risk factors apply to you, discuss them with your doctor. The two of you can develop a prevention strategy that's both practical and achievable. Women at increased risk of the disease should take action before they reach menopause. However, even if you're past menopause, you can still take positive steps to slow bone loss.

Risk factors you can't change

Some risk factors for osteoporosis you can't control. You were born with them, inherited them from your parents, or they're simply an inherent part of living. But you can take steps to slow the disease's development, and you can monitor your bone health for early signs of abnormal bone loss. These are common risk factors for the disease.

Sex

Eighty percent of all Americans with osteoporosis are women. Peak bone mass in women is usually lower than in men because women's skeletons often are smaller. Women also tend to live longer. So, in effect, women have less bone to lose and more time in which to lose it. In addition, when menopause occurs, women experience a drop in their estrogen levels, which accelerates bone loss.

Young adult men generally have 25 percent more bone mass in their vertebrae than do females of a similar age. And not surprisingly, bone mass of the male hipbone tends to be greater than that of the female hipbone.

Women are about three times as likely as men are to break a bone due to osteoporosis, and fracturing generally starts at a younger age. For example, a 50-year-old woman has a 16 percent lifetime risk of a spinal fracture whereas a 50-year-old man has a 5 percent lifetime risk. With increasing age, however, the risk begins to even out.

Age

The older you are — male or female — the more likely you are to develop osteoporosis and the more likely you are to break a bone because of it. Approximately half of women in their 80s have the disease. For more information on how aging affects bone health, see Chapter 1.

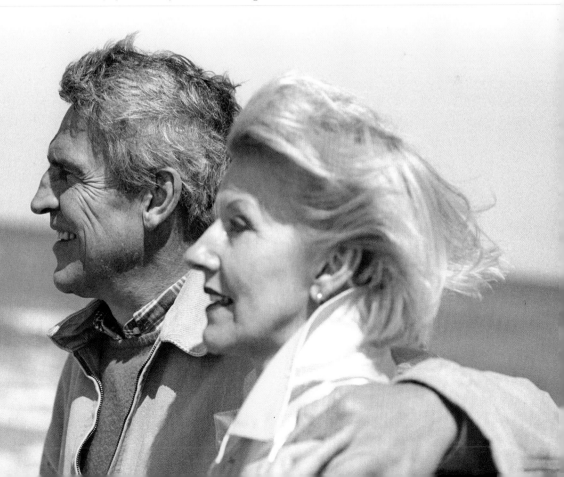

Heredity

Family history is a strong predictor of low bone mass, but it's not a very good predictor of your chances of experiencing a fracture because of osteoporosis. Studies show that genetic factors account for many differences in bone size, bone mass and bone density.

If your mother, sister, grandmother or aunt has osteoporosis, you're more likely to get it. Research also shows that if you're a woman whose mother broke her hip, you're twice as likely to break a hip, compared with the general population of women.

Several genes affect your risk of osteoporosis. These genes play a role in the density of your bones at peak bone mass as well as how rapidly you lose bone mass later in life. You also have genes that determine at what age you go through menopause and genes that regulate hormones and growth factors, all of which influence bone formation and breakdown. Other genes affect how your body uses calcium and vitamin D or how it makes the protein collagen, an essential ingredient of bone.

But your genes don't necessarily determine your bone density. Just because your mother developed osteoporosis doesn't automatically mean that the same thing will happen to you. By taking specific steps to lower your risk, you may avoid a similar fate.

Race

You're at greatest risk of osteoporosis if you're white or of Asian descent. White women past menopause experience the majority of hip fractures. Blacks have the lowest risk of osteoporosis, and Hispanics and American Indians appear to have an intermediate risk.

The various levels of risk are based in part on racial differences in bone mass and bone density. And some Asian women, for example, tend to get less calcium from their diet.

Body size

Your build also affects your risk. Petite women with a thin-boned frame are at greater risk of osteoporosis than are larger women with a thick-boned frame. This is because women who are petite and thin boned often have less bone mass to begin with, causing them to reach a fracture-prone stage at an earlier age.

Hormones

The greater your exposure to the hormone estrogen over your lifetime, the lower your risk of osteoporosis.

This means women who began menstruating later — after age 16 — don't have the bone-building effects of estrogen for as many years as women who start menstruating at an earlier age. Likewise, women who reach menopause early — either naturally in their late 40s or due to surgery before age 45 — lose the bone-building benefits of estrogen earlier than do women who experience menopause at a later age. In addition, any woman who's had her ovaries removed at an early age has a greatly increased risk of osteoporosis.

In men, a delayed onset of puberty — after age 16 — can shorten their lifetime exposure to the bone-building hormone testosterone and lower their peak bone mass. A low testosterone level during adult years can accelerate bone loss. Low estrogen levels in men (yes, men produce estrogen, too) also have been shown to be an important factor in bone loss among older men.

Men and women may also experience a reduction in testosterone and estrogen levels during certain cancer treatments.

Risk factors you can influence

Your individual circumstances or certain decisions that you make may modify your osteoporosis risk. In addition, many forms of secondary osteoporosis are treatable, or they may occur only for a certain period of time. Often times, there are steps you can take to reduce your risk of the disease.

Childbearing

Pregnancy builds stronger bones in women by raising their estrogen levels and increasing their weight. Both are beneficial to bone mass. In assessing your osteoporosis risk, your doctor will likely consider whether you've been pregnant and had children, and how many pregnancies you've had.

Remember that during pregnancy, you may experience a reduction in calcium because you're sharing your calcium supply with your baby. Breast-feeding also can drain calcium from your body. Your intestinal tract and kidneys compensate for the extra demand by absorbing and conserving more calcium. Still, if you're pregnant, make sure you're getting sufficient calcium.

Medications

Certain medications are known to accelerate bone loss and increase your risk of osteoporosis. These medicines may cause a form of secondary osteoporosis, or they may aggravate osteoporosis caused by aging or menopause. If you take these medications, talk to your doctor about what you can do to counteract their effects on your bones.

Corticosteroid medicines

Long-term use of corticosteroids such as prednisone, cortisone, prednisolone and dexamethasone is especially damaging to bone. These medications, also called glucocorticoids, are commonly used to treat asthma, rheumatoid arthritis and other inflammatory conditions. They lower bone mass by slowing bone formation and by decreasing your blood levels of estrogen and testosterone.

Any dosage of an oral or intravenous corticosteroid increases your risk of fracture. However, these drugs are prescribed because of their benefits. If your doctor has you taking one of these medications, he or she has good reasons for doing so. Don't stop taking it, and don't change your dose without first talking to your doctor. If you take the medicine for more than a few weeks, it's likely that your doctor will monitor your bone density and recommend drugs that prevent bone loss.

Inhaled corticosteroids may cause a small amount of bone loss in the lumbar spine. Corticosteroids taken in nasal spray form haven't been shown to result in bone loss.

Anticonvulsants

Medications taken to control seizures include the drugs phenobarbital, phenytoin (Dilantin), carbamazepine (Carbatrol, Tegretol) and valproic acid (Depakene). If this type of medication is used over a long period of time, your liver starts to metabolize vitamin D in a way that causes a deficiency of the vitamin. If you take one of these medications, your doctor may recommend vitamin D and calcium supplements.

Thyroid medicines

If used in excessive quantities, thyroid medications such as levothyroxine (Levothroid, Levoxyl, Synthroid) can cause hyperthyroidism, leading to accelerated bone loss. Because your requirements for thyroid hormone can change over time, a blood test for thyroid-stimulating hormone (TSH) should be done annually. The test determines if you're taking the right amount of medicine. The dose can be adjusted if necessary.

Diuretics

Diuretics are drugs that prevent fluid buildup in your body. In so doing, certain diuretics may cause your kidneys to excrete too much calcium. If you're not getting enough calcium and other bone-building minerals in your diet, you may experience bone loss.

Diuretics that may cause this problem include bumetanide (Bumex), furosemide (Lasix), ethacrynic acid (Edecrin) and torsemide (Demadex). Other diuretics, called thiazides, may actually help your body retain calcium. Always talk to your doctor about any risks associated with your medications. You may be able to switch to a diuretic that doesn't cause calcium loss.

Other medications

Other medications that can increase the risk of osteoporosis include:

Blood thinners. Blood thinners are prescribed to prevent blood clots from developing in your veins and arteries. Low molecular weight heparin, which is widely used to prevent blood clots, isn't associated with bone loss. However, traditional heparin may cause bone loss if used over long periods of time. Newer blood thinners, such as the drug dabigatran (Pradaxa), haven't been shown to cause bone loss.

Gonadotrophin-releasing hormone agonists. This is a class of drugs used to suppress blood levels of estrogen and testosterone. It includes the medications leuprolide acetate (Lupron, Viadur) and nafarelin (Synarel). These drugs are effective in treating conditions such as endometriosis, severe premenstrual syndrome (PMS) and prostate cancer. Reduced levels of estrogen and testosterone can also result in rapid bone loss. Levels usually return to normal after the dosage is stopped.

Aromatase inhibitors. Aromatase inhibitors are newer medications used to treat breast cancer. They include the medications exemestane (Aromasin), letrozole (Femara) and anastrozole (Arimidex). Aromatase inhibitors speed up loss of bone mass, increasing your risk of a fracture.

Medical conditions

Certain medical conditions can increase your risk of osteoporosis by slowing bone formation or speeding up bone resorption. Some of these conditions may cause a form of secondary osteoporosis.

Endocrine disorders
Your endocrine system produces hormones that help regulate many body activities and functions. Problems with endocrine glands associated with bone growth and maintenance can disrupt your bone remodeling cycle.

Hypogonadism. This condition occurs from a lack of estrogen and testosterone, leading to abnormal bone loss. Many factors can affect hormone production, including certain medications, various diseases of the ovaries or testes, natural aging, and eating disorders that disrupt menstruation.

Hyperparathyroidism. This is the result of overactive glands supplying too much parathyroid hormone (PTH) to your bloodstream. Too much PTH may result in release of too much calcium from your bones and increase your risk of fracture.

Cushing's syndrome. Cushing's syndrome occurs when the adrenal glands produce too much cortisol, a corticosteroid that slows bone formation and can increase bone resorption.

Diabetes. Type 1 diabetes, which must be treated with insulin, is associated with bone loss, especially if the condition is poorly controlled. People with type 2 diabetes, the more common form, may also be at higher risk of bone fracture.

Gastrointestinal disorders

Some gastrointestinal diseases can affect the bone remodeling cycle and lead to bone loss. They do so by interfering with the way your intestines absorb calcium from the food you eat and by lowering your vitamin D level.

Intestinal disorders. Disorders of the small intestine that interfere with absorption of calcium and vitamin D, such as Crohn's disease and celiac disease, can result in reduced bone mass. Sometimes these conditions are treated with a corticosteroid medication, which further inhibits calcium absorption and vitamin D levels.

Liver disorders. Certain disorders of the liver are rare but notorious for causing osteoporosis. Primary biliary cirrhosis occurs when tiny bile ducts in the liver become inflamed and scarred. This disorder occurs most often among women between the ages of 35 and 60.

Lactose intolerance. This condition causes gas, stomach cramps and diarrhea when you consume dairy products containing milk sugar (lactose). If you're lactose intolerant or you don't consume dairy products for other reasons, it's important to take calcium supplements or eat plenty of nondairy foods high in calcium.

Rheumatoid arthritis

Rheumatoid arthritis is an inflammatory condition that causes painful aching and swelling in your joints. The disease appears to be triggered by an abnormal response from your body's immune system. Therefore, it's referred to as an autoimmune disease. The principal area of attack of rheumatoid arthritis is the lining of your joints, leading to the gradual destruction of cartilage, bone, tendons and ligaments in the joint. The condition can keep people from being physically active, increasing their risk of bone loss. It may also be treated with corticosteroids and other medications that can damage bone.

Amenorrhea

Absent or irregular menstrual cycles in women of childbearing age may be a sign of low estrogen levels. Amenorrhea may result from eating or malabsorption disorders, excessive exercise, or disorders of the ovaries or pituitary gland. If you have a history of abnormal menstrual cycles, your risk of osteoporosis is increased.

Surgical procedures

Organ transplants can result in bone loss because the immunosuppressant medications you generally have to take afterward may interfere with bone formation. This includes corticosteroid medications, known to damage bone.

Gastric surgery to remove part of your stomach can cause bone loss because you're less able to absorb calcium and vitamin D from your food. Intestinal bypass surgery and certain bariatric surgeries for weight loss also can result in osteoporosis. The part of the intestine where many minerals and vitamins are easily absorbed is bypassed, so the body doesn't absorb iron, calcium and other nutrients as efficiently, increasing your risk of osteoporosis.

Prolonged bed rest

If you're on prolonged bed rest or are immobilized because of stroke, fracture, surgery or paralysis, consult your doctor regarding what you can do to prevent abnormal bone loss.

Risk factors you can change

Some risk factors that put you at risk of osteoporosis you can control. That means you may be able to eliminate them or at least greatly reduce their effect on your skeleton. Osteoporosis is easier to prevent than it is to treat. That's why it's important to understand those risk factors over which you have control — those you can change.

Weight and dieting

Eating disorders and obesity can affect your bone health and your risk of osteoporosis. Your goal is not to weigh too much or too little, but to maintain a healthy weight.

Obesity. Obesity was once thought to protect against bone loss, but researchers are no longer certain that is the case. Recent studies suggest that some people who are obese have hidden fat inside their bone marrow. The fat is thought to take up space where cells responsible for new bone formation reside. The belief is that with less new bone being formed, existing bone becomes weakened and more prone to fracture. Additional research is needed to more fully explore the relationship between excess weight and osteoporosis.

Eating disorders. In our weight-obsessed society, you may try to stay thin by keeping food off your plate. But if you starve your body, you also starve

Risk evaluation for osteoporosis

Answering these questions can help you evaluate your risk of osteoporosis. The more yes answers you have, the higher your risk.

	Yes	No
• Are you female?	❑	❑
• Have you stopped menstruating?	❑	❑
• Have you ever broken a bone?	❑	❑
• Have you experienced a loss of height?	❑	❑
• Do you have a family history of osteoporosis?	❑	❑
• Are you white or Asian?	❑	❑
• Are you petite or small boned?	❑	❑
• Did you start menstruation at age 16 or older?	❑	❑
• Did you have irregular periods before menopause?	❑	❑
• Were you never pregnant?	❑	❑
• Did you go through menopause before age 45?	❑	❑
• Have you taken medication for a year or more that could increase bone loss?	❑	❑
• Have you ever had a medical condition that's known to increase your risk of osteoporosis?	❑	❑
• Do you include little or no foods containing calcium in your diet?	❑	❑
• Have you dieted frequently or ever lost an excessive amount of weight?	❑	❑
• Do you not exercise?	❑	❑
• Do you smoke tobacco products?	❑	❑
• Do you drink more than 2 ounces of alcohol each day?	❑	❑

your bones. Serious eating disorders such as anorexia nervosa and bulimia can damage your skeleton by depriving your body of essential nutrients needed for bone building and maintenance.

Anorexia nervosa is an eating disorder triggered by an overwhelming fear of weight gain. It primarily affects young women — lowering their estrogen levels during an important time of skeletal development. A person with anorexia nervosa may begin losing bone at an earlier age and lose bone more rapidly than normal.

In addition to eating disorders, bone health may be affected by excessive dieting. Your peak bone mass, which you achieve in your young adult years, is influenced by your weight. Thin women tend to produce less estrogen — the hormone that builds bone — and heavier women tend to produce more. Women who lose significant weight through dieting may lose bone mass as well. Bariatric surgery for weight loss also can reduce bone density.

The best approach for your bones — and your overall health — is to keep your weight within a normal range for your age and your height. And if you do diet, do it in a healthy manner, taking steps to preserve bone density.

Physical activity

Use your bones or lose your bones. Regular activity and exercise are keys to preventing osteoporosis and fractures. Children who are the most physically active often have a high bone density and reach a higher peak bone mass than do children who don't get enough exercise.

Lack of physical activity also accelerates bone loss when you're older. Studies show that adults who sit all day at a desk job and don't exercise are more apt to lose bone mass and suffer fractures than are adults who fit some form of physical activity into their day.

Weight-bearing exercises such as walking or resistance training can increase or at least maintain your bone density at any age. For more information on appropriate activities and exercises for bone health, see Chapter 9.

Smoking

If you smoke, you already have plenty of good reasons to stop. But here's another — smoking is bad to the bone. It interferes with production of estrogen and testosterone. Smoking also disrupts calcium absorption and the bone-formation part of the remodeling cycle. That may be a reason smokers are more likely to experience osteoporosis and to have bone fractures.

Menopause, which accelerates bone loss, happens on an average of two years earlier in women who smoke than in nonsmokers. And postmenopausal smokers lose bone at a faster rate than do postmenopausal nonsmokers. Smokers also tend to drink more alcohol and not exercise or eat as healthy as nonsmokers. These behaviors increase your risk of osteoporosis. The good news is, even if you're older, if you stop smoking right now, you can slow your bone loss.

Alcohol use

Consuming too much alcohol over a long period of time can increase your risk of osteoporosis and fractures. Alcohol causes a double whammy: It's toxic to bone-building osteoblasts, and it stimulates bone-removing osteoclasts, increasing bone loss. People who drink heavily on a regular basis also have lower levels of the hormones estrogen and testosterone. More than an ounce of alcohol a day for women and 2 ounces a day for men can lead to these effects.

Vertebral fractures are uncommon in people younger than age 50, but they're more likely to be seen in individuals who drink heavily, eat poorly and don't exercise. These individuals are also more likely to fall and break a bone because alcohol impairs their balance.

People who stop drinking alcohol are often able to restore normal bone-building function and, if they're relatively young, they may even recover some lost bone mass.

Then you and your doctor can plan your strategy for lowering and even eliminating some of your risk factors. The earlier in life you do this, the better. But remember that it's never too late to start. You may wish to ask your doctor about a bone density test. You can learn all about this important test in the next chapter.

What's next?

Osteoporosis is a treatable disease, and bone fractures associated with it aren't inevitable. Taking steps to maintain strong bones and a healthy skeleton is important because your first fracture greatly increases your risk of future fractures.

Now that you've had a chance to review those factors that can increase or decrease your risk of osteoporosis and bone fractures, you may wish to discuss them with your doctor. Together you can determine whether you're at high, moderate or low risk. Generally, being at high risk means you have two or more risk factors.

Chapter 5

Screening and diagnosis

How do you know if you have osteoporosis or are at risk? This is a common question, and one you may want answered sooner rather than later. The sooner you can start on prevention strategies, the better your chances of keeping your skeleton healthy. And if you already have osteoporosis, the earlier you treat it, the better your chances of slowing bone loss and stabilizing your condition.

It used to be the only way to detect osteoporosis was when you broke a bone. Things are different now. A bone density test, also known as bone densitometry, can determine if you have osteoporosis before any bones are broken. It can also detect if your bone density is lower than normal for a person of your age and sex. Decreased bone density that's likely to progress to osteoporosis

without treatment or other preventive measures is known as osteopenia.

In addition to having you undergo a bone density test, your doctor can learn much about your bone health from a thorough health history and physical examination. These evaluations can help identify secondary causes of osteoporosis. Other tests also may be done.

Screening vs. diagnosing

Before delving into the details of tests that help determine your bone health, it's important that you're clear on the distinction between screening tests and diagnostic tests.

Screening tests

Screening tests are tests that are done on someone who has no apparent signs or symptoms of a disease. If the test result registers as abnormal, it may reveal the presence of a previously unsuspected problem.

Screening tests tend to be less sensitive — but also less expensive — than diagnostic tests. You may undergo a screening test for osteoporosis if you have certain risk factors for the disease but you don't have any apparent signs or symptoms. For example, you may be a middle-aged woman with a family history of osteoporosis, but you haven't experienced a broken bone, loss of height or sudden-onset back pain.

You should consider being screened for osteoporosis at least once during your lifetime. Be aware, though, that there's some controversy among doctors as to exactly when a screening test should be done.

The test used to check your bone density is called bone densitometry. You don't need a referral from your doctor to have the test. You can have it done at a community health fair or other similar setting. If the results suggest your bones are weaker than they should be

for someone your age and sex, contact your doctor for more in-depth testing.

Diagnostic tests

Diagnostic tests are performed on someone who's suspected of having a disorder, such as osteoporosis, because of certain risk factors or the presence of signs or symptoms.

Diagnostic tests are generally more precise and more expensive than are screening tests. If you're age 40 or older and you break a bone, you may undergo diagnostic testing for osteoporosis. The primary diagnostic test is a bone density test, accompanied by a medical history and physical examination. You'll learn later in this chapter why a history and physical evaluation are important for making a diagnosis.

The results of diagnostic tests can help:

- Confirm you have osteoporosis
- Determine its severity
- Establish baseline bone density value

Testing is generally arranged by your doctor and done with a more accurate device than what is used for most screening tests.

What's a bone density test?

A bone density test is about as close as your doctor can come to predicting your future bone health. From test results, he or she can tell if you have osteoporosis and give you a good indication of how susceptible your bones are to fracture.

The test is simple, fast and painless. It uses special X-rays to measure how many grams of calcium and other bone minerals (bone mineral content) are packed into a square centimeter of bone. A gram is about $1/28$ of an ounce. A centimeter is about half an inch.

The terms *bone mineral content* and *bone density* are often used interchangeably. Here's why: Generally the higher your mineral content, the denser your bones. And the denser your bones, the less likely they are to fracture.

Bone density tests are usually done on bones that are most likely to break if you have osteoporosis. These sites include the lumbar vertebrae located in your lower spine, the narrow neck of your femur bone near where the bone adjoins the hip, and the bones of your wrist or forearm.

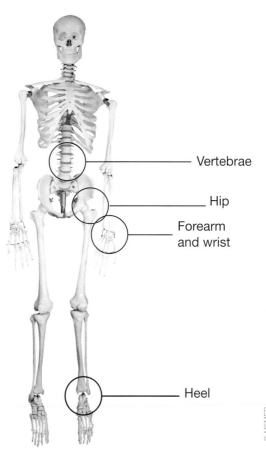

© MFMER

Common fracture sites Bone density testing may occur in one or more of these locations.

Who should be tested?

Adults at risk of osteoporosis should have their bone density measured. Early testing makes it possible to begin preventive measures and give them time to work. Testing is also the first step toward diagnosis and treatment.

It's generally recommended that all women have their bones checked at least once during their lifetimes. A bone density test is also recommended for the following individuals:

- All women age 65 and older
- Postmenopausal women younger than 65 years who have two or more risk factors for the disease
- Men age 70 and older at risk of osteoporosis
- Anyone older than age 40 who breaks a bone in a nontraumatic event from a fall at standing height or less (fragility fracture)
- Anyone receiving ongoing treatment with glucocorticoids
- Anyone with a low estrogen or testosterone level (hypogonadism)
- Any woman, man or child at high risk of bone loss and fracture

Instead of waiting until age 65, many women have a bone density test at menopause, even if they have no risk factors. An earlier test is especially advisable if you're at high risk of osteoporosis or if you've broken a bone or have experienced a loss in height.

Any woman past menopause who breaks a bone should be tested because osteoporosis may be responsible for causing the fracture. If osteoporosis is the cause, the test can determine the severity of the disease.

Bone density testing usually isn't a one-time event. Bone density tests taken at intervals over several years can reveal the rate at which you're losing bone. The rate of bone loss is a potent predictor of your fracture risk.

How often you should be retested is often determined by the results of your first test. A recent study funded by the National Institutes of Health concluded that individuals with osteoporosis should be retested in a year, and those who don't have osteoporosis can wait several years to be retested. Your doctor will also take into consideration changes to your health, a change in medications, and other risk factors that may increase your risk and warrant earlier testing.

How often to have a bone density test

Results of first test	When to retest
Normal	17 years
Osteopenia	5 years
Osteoporosis	1 year

© *New England Journal of Medicine* 2012; 366:225.

What does bone density tell you?

A bone density test provides a snapshot of the mineral content of a section of bone at a single moment in time. This snapshot can:

- Determine if you have low bone density in specific parts of your skeleton
- Determine if you have osteoporosis

If you're tested at intervals of a year or more, the results can be compared and used to:

- Identify changes in bone density that may be occurring over time
- Determine how your bone density is responding to treatment

If you're taking medicine to treat osteoporosis, you may benefit from annual testing the first couple of years until it's clear that your bone mass is stable or improving. Thereafter, the tests can be less frequent. If you're taking corticosteroids, it's recommended that you be tested once a year.

Only a small fraction of adults who have osteoporosis or are at risk are properly screened, diagnosed and treated. Part of the reason is that not enough people get bone density tests. One study of 34,000 women older than age 50 found very few of the women had ever had a bone density test. This was in spite of the fact that almost half of them had one or more risk factors for the disease.

How do you get tested?

Perhaps the best way to arrange a bone density test is through your primary care doctor. If during your routine physical exam your doctor doesn't suggest a bone density test, it may be up to you to call it to his or her attention. Don't be shy about inquiring about a test, particularly if you've broken a bone, are nearing menopause or simply want to be screened.

Most tests take place in hospitals, usually in the radiology department. Some hospitals have special osteoporosis programs, often as part of a women's health center. Some larger cities even have osteoporosis centers unaffiliated with a hospital. If you don't have a personal physician, a hospital in your community can direct you to where you can be tested.

Endocrinologists — doctors who specialize in the body's hormonal system — are specially trained to screen, diagnose and treat osteoporosis. However, other types of medical specialists, such as rheumatologists, may have osteoporosis training as well.

Keep in mind that bone density testing that involves portable devices set up in drugstores or at community health fairs is generally less accurate than the testing done in medical centers.

Who pays for testing?

Depending on where you get tested and what type of device is used, some health insurance plans pay for the test and others don't. You may need to ask your health plan administrator if bone density testing is covered under your plan and how much of the cost is paid.

Private insurance plans often follow Medicare guidelines regarding payment. Coverage may also depend on whether the procedure is labeled a screening or diagnostic test. The test is often considered a screening test if you have no signs or symptoms and the results show you don't have osteoporosis. If you have signs or symptoms, the test is usually considered diagnostic.

How testing is done

Bone density testing uses a device called a bone densitometer. Most densitometers measure the absorption of a low-energy X-ray beam as it passes through bone, in comparison to the absorption of the X-ray beam as it passes through the soft tissues next to the bone. The amount of X-ray energy (photons) that enters the bone is also compared with the amount of energy that leaves the bone. The denser the bone, the more of the X-ray beam that's absorbed.

Why not use regular X-rays for a bone density test? Regular X-rays are higher energy and optimal for a wide variety of imaging. But the energy of regular X-rays isn't sensitive enough to detect low bone density until a bone has lost 25 to 40 percent of its mineral content. By then osteoporosis may already be in an advanced stage.

Government assistance for bone density testing

Medicare and Medicaid pay for bone density tests under specific circumstances. How much they pay varies, depending on where you live.

Medicare. Medicare is the federal health insurance program for individuals age 65 and older who receive Social Security benefits. At the present time, the program pays for bone density tests on all people age 65 and older at risk of osteoporosis who meet the following criteria:

- A women whose doctor determines she's estrogen deficient and at risk of osteoporosis, based on her medical history and other findings
- A person whose X-rays show possible osteoporosis, osteopenia or vertebral fractures
- A person taking prednisone or steroid-type medications, or who will soon begin such treatment
- A person who's been diagnosed with primary hyperparathyroidism
- A person who's being monitored to see if medication to treat osteoporosis is working

For more information, visit the Medicare website: *www.medicare.gov*.

Medicaid. Medicaid is a federal program that helps pay medical costs for low-income Americans and people with certain disabilities. It's known in some states as medical assistance. This program is administered by each state's individual welfare system, so the benefits and eligibility requirements vary from state to state.

For more information, contact the accounts payable department at your local medical clinic or a social service agency within your state government. You can also visit the Centers for Medicare & Medicaid Services website at *www.cms.gov*.

Radiation exposure from X-ray beams used in bone density testing is very low — only a fraction of the radiation used for a standard chest X-ray. You don't need to wear a protective apron, and the person testing you doesn't need to leave the room.

All bone density tests are quick, painless and noninvasive. The tests usually take about 10 to 15 minutes, depending on the type of densitometer being used. This doesn't include the time needed for filling out forms and other preparation work.

A radiologist, endocrinologist or other bone specialist will assess your test results. If the results indicate you have bone loss, you'll likely be prescribed a treatment plan to slow or stop the loss. The type of treatment you receive will depend on a variety of factors, including the cause of your osteoporosis.

Types of bone densitometers

Densitometers come in several sizes and their levels of accuracy also vary. Some types work better on specific bones than do others.

Central densitometers

Central densitometers are relatively large — large enough for you to lie down on — and they're usually found in medical centers or hospitals. As the name suggests, these instruments are used to measure the density of the central, stabilizing parts of your skeleton, such as the spine and hip. But they can also be used on any bone in the body.

Central densitometers provide the most accurate bone density tests and are good predictors of your potential risk of fracture. There are two types of central densitometers: dual energy X-ray absorptiometry and quantitative computerized tomography.

Dual energy X-ray absorptiometry (DXA)

A DXA test is the most accurate way to measure your bone density. That's why doctors typically rely on this test to diagnose osteoporosis. A DXA machine uses two different X-ray beams, which increases the precision of the measurement. A DXA test can detect as little as a 3 to 5 percent change in bone density between successive scans.

To begin the test, you lie down on a padded platform. Once you're in position, mechanical arms that contain an X-ray source (located under the table) and an X-ray detector (located above your body) are properly aligned. The amount of X-ray energy absorbed by the bone is measured to determine your bone density. The healthier your bone is, the less X-ray energy that passes through it. With the latest equipment, a DXA test takes only a few minutes to obtain an accurate result.

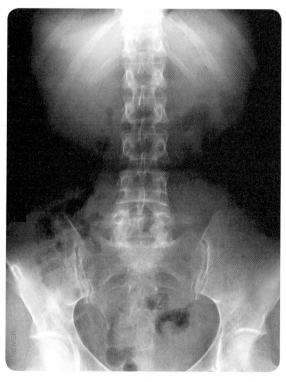

A look inside Bones of different densities will appear differently on an X-ray image. This image of the pelvis and spine shows areas of denser bone (lighter areas) and more porous bone (darker areas).

DXA is most often performed on the narrow neck of your femur bone, just below the hip joint, as well as the lumbar vertebrae, which form the lower portion of your spine. The narrow neck of the femur is a good predictor of your risk of hip fracture, which is the most serious complication of osteoporosis. A DXA test of the hip is often used to predict future fracture risk of other bones as well.

Because of its accuracy, DXA is the preferred test for a baseline bone density measurement for anyone starting medication to treat osteoporosis.

Quantitative computerized tomography (QCT)

This procedure measures your bone density using computerized tomography (CT). Similar to having a CT scan, you lie on a movable padded table that slides into a large ring where the measurements are made. X-ray images are obtained from all angles. Special bone density computer software processes these images and combines them into a single scan that's useful for assessing bone structure. The test usually takes about 10 minutes.

QCT is most often used to measure density in your vertebrae and the portion of the femur bone below your hip.

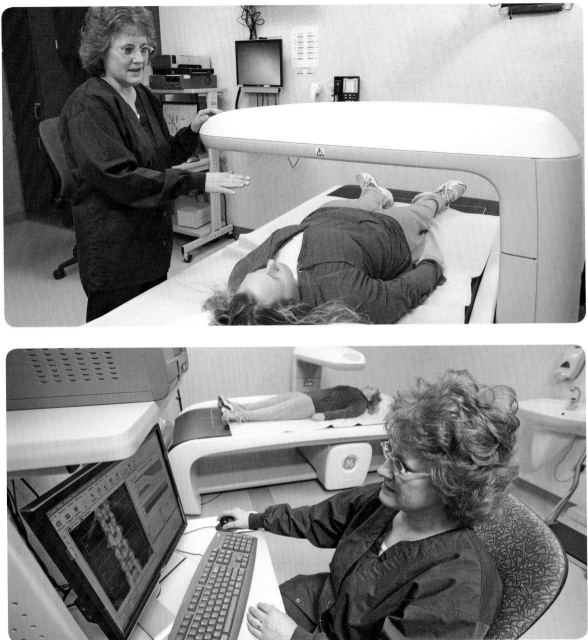

DXA test Dual energy X-ray absorptiometry (DXA) is the most accurate procedure to diagnose osteoporosis. This set of photos shows a DXA scan of the spine. The woman lies flat on her back and the arm of the device is positioned over her spine (top). The arm measures her bone density by detecting energy from an X-ray source located under the table. The information is transmitted to a computer, where an image of the woman's spine appears, along with a summary of her bone density measurements (bottom).

Bone scans and bone biopsies

Bone density tests aren't the same as bone scans or bone biopsies. Bone scans often are used to diagnose cancer or occasionally a rare bone disease. A small amount of radioactive dye is injected into your bloodstream where it collects in your bones. This allows a radiologist to see problem hot spots. Much as with a bone density test, your body's exposure to radiation from a bone scan is very small.

A bone biopsy is a procedure that uses a hollow needle to remove a small sample of bone tissue from your hip. This sample is tested to see if you have other bone diseases, such as osteomalacia, which is a softening of bone caused by a variety of conditions. A bone biopsy can also be useful in determining bone disease associated with kidney failure.

Test results may be used to monitor how well you're responding to treatment. A QCT test is more expensive than are other densitometry tests and exposes you to more radiation.

Peripheral densitometers

Peripheral densitometers are smaller and less expensive than central densitometers. They're used to measure bone density on the periphery of your skeleton, such as in your wrist and heel bones. Peripheral densitometers aren't as accurate as the central devices in predicting your risk of hip fracture, but they're accurate enough to screen anyone at risk of osteoporosis.

You can find peripheral devices in some drugstores and other retail locations set up for do-it-yourself use. This type of test is often offered free or for only a few dollars as part of a health fair or store promotion.

If the results of a peripheral test show that you have low bone density, you'll want to follow that up with a central densitometer test. It provides a more accurate result and can help you and your doctor determine what measures are necessary to either prevent or treat the condition. Several types of peripheral densitometry tests are available:

Quantitative ultrasound (QUS)

This procedure is often called heel ultrasound because most often it measures bone density in the heel bone. Instead of X-ray radiation, QUS sends high-frequency sound waves through your heel while you rest your bare foot on the instrument. And rather than measure X-ray absorption, this type of densitometer measures the reflection of sound waves. The denser your bone, the sooner sound waves are reflected back to the device.

This type of densitometer is portable, low cost and widely available. It measures your bone density in less than a minute. QUS is an easy way to be screened if you think you're at risk of osteoporosis. However, it's not accurate enough to positively diagnose osteoporosis or osteopenia — bone density that's below normal and likely to progress to osteoporosis without some type of intervention.

Heel ultrasound is almost as accurate as DXA at predicting your risk of breaking a hip or an arm or wrist. But it can't measure changes in your central skeleton over time or tell if your bones are responding to medication. In addi-

tion, because the heel bone is subjected to constant pressure from bearing the weight of your upper body, it's generally not considered the best location to test for certain types of bone mineral changes.

Peripheral dual energy X-ray absorptiometry (pDXA)

This test uses a compact, portable DXA scanner. With the use of X-rays, pDXA measures bone density in your wrist or heel. The test takes about three minutes and is accurate enough to screen anyone at risk of osteoporosis. Because pDXA is more expensive than a QUS test and the device is less portable, it isn't used as often as QUS.

Peripheral quantitative computerized tomography (pQCT)

This test also is rarely used because it's more expensive than similar screening examinations. In addition, it produces a higher radiation exposure than do other tests.

The test utilizes a small, portable QCT machine that measures the bone density of your wrist or hand. While seated with your hand, wrist or forearm placed inside the machine, X-rays pass through your bone, and the machine calculates your bone density. The procedure takes about 10 minutes.

Types of bone densitometers

Technique	Abbreviation	Common testing location
Central		
Dual energy X-ray absorptiometry	DXA	Spine, hip, forearm and total body
Quantitative computerized tomography	QCT	Spine and hip
Peripheral		
Quantitative ultrasound	QUS	Heel
Peripheral dual energy X-ray absorptiometry	pDXA	Wrist or heel
Peripheral quantitative computerized tomography	pQCT	Wrist or hand
High-resolution peripheral quantitative computerized tomography	HRpQCT	Forearm or lower leg
High-resolution MRI	micro-MRI	Wrist, ankle or heel

High-resolution pQCT (HRpQCT)

Also known as 3DpQCT or XtremeCT, this sophisticated technology assesses bone microstructure in addition to bone density using three dimensional imaging. HRpQCT measures bone strength and quality in the forearm and lower leg. The test, which is currently undergoing evaluation, is thought to provide better insight into bone health than devices more commonly used today.

High-resolution magnetic resonance imaging (micro-MRI)

Another investigational technology, this device is used at peripheral sites, such as the wrist, ankle and heel. Think of it as a micro-MRI machine. It can assess bone micro-structure and strength with the use of stronger magnetic fields and new types of technology. Like HRpQCT, the device is undergoing study and isn't commonly used.

Which test is right for you?

The type of bone density test that's best for you depends on your age and on why you're being tested. Perhaps you're worried because you have risk factors that make you susceptible to osteoporosis. Maybe you're concerned about a particular bone. Or maybe you have no risk factors but are simply curious about the health of your bones.

If you haven't had a bone density test yet, but you would like to have one to learn more about the health of your bones, here's some information that can help you decide which test is best in your situation.

You have no risk factors

If you don't have any risk factors for osteoporosis and you haven't broken a bone, a less expensive peripheral screening test, such as a pDXA or QUS, may be sufficient. If the results indicate low bone density, you and your doctor will likely want to follow up with tests from a more accurate central densitometer, such as a DXA.

If you're worried about the strength of a specific bone, be tested with the device that most accurately measures that part of your skeleton. Your doctor can advise you.

You have multiple risk factors or a broken bone

If you suspect that you may have osteoporosis, your doctor can arrange for a DXA test — even if the result of an earlier peripheral test was normal. A woman younger than age 65 is more likely to experience a vertebral fracture than a hip fracture, so a DXA of the spine may be the most accurate indicator. Just the opposite, in women age 65 and older, hip fractures are increasingly common, so a DXA of the hip may reveal more.

DXA can measure bone density accurately in other parts of your skeleton. That's good because osteoporosis tends to affect different parts of your skeleton at different times. In addition, different parts of a skeleton lose bone at different rates, particularly in postmenopausal women. For these reasons, it's often a good idea to test more than one location. Your bone density may be normal at one site but low at another.

You suspect secondary osteoporosis

A disease, surgical procedure or certain medications can result in secondary osteoporosis, bone loss that's triggered by another medical condition. Your doctor will select a testing procedure based on what he or she thinks may be causing your bone loss.

If, for example, you have hyperpara-thyroidism, you may be losing mostly cortical bone, in which case a DXA of your forearm may be the best choice because your forearm is made mostly of cortical bone.

You have osteoporosis

If you have osteoporosis, your doctor may schedule periodic DXA tests of the primary fracture sites — your hip, spine, wrist or a combination of these. When testing is performed regularly, it's recommended that the same machine (densitometer) be used each time, as well as the same technician. And, of course, the testing should be performed on the same bone. These steps will help produce the most accurate results.

The reason your doctor may recommend this is because test results are slightly different for each machine. Densitometry experts are working on a way to compare test results from different densitometers.

You're monitoring your treatment

If you're taking medication for osteo-porosis, central densitometry of your spine is best. The trabecular bone in your spine best shows the effects of medication. Peripheral densitometry isn't accurate enough to provide this type of information.

History and physical exam

Many people mistakenly believe that a bone density test is all you need to diagnose osteoporosis. It's true the test can confirm that you have low bone density, but it can't tell you why. Is something about your general health or lifestyle damaging your bones? To answer this question, you'll need a complete medical evaluation, including a medical history and physical exam.

To get a medical history, your doctor will ask you questions about your personal health history and the medical history of your close relatives. You also may be asked about medications you're taking, what you eat, how much you exercise, and how much tobacco and alcohol you use. Be honest with your answers. Your doctor isn't there to judge you but to determine your risk of osteoporosis and to identify other conditions that may cause the symptoms.

A physical exam involves common medical tests, such as checking your blood pressure and heart rate. You may also have blood and urine tests. Combined with your medical history, a physical evaluation helps your doctor interpret the results of your bone density test.

Bone marker tests

Bone marker tests measure bone turnover, that is, the rate at which bone changes. Test results don't indicate in which direction the remodeling cycle is headed — whether you're losing more bone or growing more — only that there's a change. Because these results aren't always the type of information your doctor needs to understand your bone health, marker tests are used less often than bone density tests in diagnosis and treatment.

Here's how a bone marker test works. The bone remodeling cycle releases chemical byproducts into your bloodstream and urine. These byproducts are remnants of the materials that make up your bone as well as hormones and enzymes associated with the remodeling cycle. A blood or urine sample can indicate the rate at which bone breakdown (resorption) and formation are occurring. If it's known that you're losing bone at the time a bone marker test is given, a high rate of bone turnover means faster bone loss.

Bone marker tests can't be used to diagnose osteoporosis, and they aren't used in the day-to-day management of the condition.

Who should have a bone marker test?

Bone marker tests generally aren't good at predicting fracture risk, although sometimes they can be used when the results are compared with a bone density test of the hip.

You may not need a bone marker test if you have the most common types of osteoporosis, which are associated with aging and menopause. Bone marker tests are most useful if your bone loss is associated with a medical condition whose effect on your skeleton isn't known. The results can indicate if the condition is affecting bone turnover.

Bone marker tests are also useful in monitoring treatment for osteoporosis. It often takes one to two years of drug treatment before significant changes in bone density can be measured. That's a long time to wait to find out if your treatment is working. Bone marker tests, meanwhile, can indicate if drug therapy is producing positive results in as little as three to six months.

Types

Some bone marker tests measure byproducts of bone formation, and others measure byproducts of bone breakdown. Some measure byproducts in your urine, and others measure them in your blood.

Bone marker tests cause minimal or no pain. But many factors — including your diet, the time of day that the test is administered and, in women, the menstrual cycle — can influence the tests and limit their usefulness. Blood (serum) tests are generally preferred over urine tests because they produce less variable results and, therefore, are more reliable.

Bone marker tests are divided into two groups — resorption markers and formation markers.

Resorption markers
These tests measure byproducts of bone breakdown. They include:

Serum CTx-telopeptide (CTx). This test measures a compound released into the bloodstream when bone is broken down. The higher the amount, the quicker bone is being resorbed. The lower the amount, the slower it's being resorbed.

Serum or urine NTx-telopeptide (NTx). This test is similar to the serum CTx test, but it measures a different compound excreted during bone resorption.

Formation markers

These tests measure byproducts of bone formation. They include:

Serum procollagen carboxy terminal extension peptide (P1NP). This test measures the rate at which new fibrous tissue (collagen) is formed within bone.

Serum bone-specific alkaline phosphatase and serum osteocalcin. These tests are similar to the P1NP test but measure different compounds.

A medical history and physical exam determine your general state of health and may help your doctor detect a possible disorder that could cause osteoporosis. Bone marker tests also may alert your doctor to a secondary cause, but these tests are generally more helpful in monitoring treatment.

After your bone density test, you'll probably have a follow-up visit with your doctor to discuss the test results. You'll get more out of that discussion if you understand what all of the numbers and lines on your printout mean. You can learn more about this in the next chapter.

Making a diagnosis

Of the tools your doctor has for diagnosing osteoporosis, a bone density test combined with a medical history and a physical exam are the most important.

A DXA scan of the hip is usually the best tool to calculate your fracture risk and, based on this information, determine if you have osteoporosis.

Chapter 6

Making sense of test results

You just had a bone density test and you get the results. Good grief! Look at all of the lines and numbers! What do they mean?

A bone density test measures the mineral content of your bones — the amount of minerals, such as calcium and phosphate, that are packed into a square centimeter of bone. Those seemingly incomprehensible numbers and lines on a computer screen or a paper printout indicate your bone mass, and they provide insight into the health of your skeleton.

Bone density isn't the only factor that determines bone strength, but it's the only factor that can be measured. Any location on your skeleton with a very low bone density measurement is at high risk of fracture. And it's not the only part of your body in jeopardy. For example, if a bone density test of your hip indicates low bone mass, not only do you have an increased chance of breaking your hip, you also have an increased chance of fracturing a vertebra.

Well-defined criteria have been developed for interpreting bone density measurements. Two numbers from the test results that draw the most attention are your T-score and your Z-score.

What's included

The results of a bone density test may not make a whole lot of sense when you first see the report. Once your doctor explains what the lines, numbers and colors represent, the report

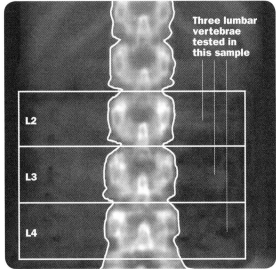

© MFMER

DXA image Main elements from a bone density test of the spine include an image of the bone being tested (above) and a summary table and graph (adjoining page). This DXA test indicates someone in his or her early 40s with good bone density of the lumbar region of the spine.

becomes a bit easier to understand. Test results usually include at least three elements:

- An image (black-and-white or color)
- A summary table of bone density numbers
- A graph

These elements are what a doctor sees on the computer screen while performing your bone density test. The image is a graphic representation of bone density. The example above shows that this

test was performed on the spine. White rectangles are superimposed over the image of three of the vertebrae. The labels L2, L3 and L4 indicate that, for this test, bone density was measured on the second, third and fourth vertebrae in the lumbar region of the spine.

The summary table that accompanies this image is located on the top of the opposite page. In the first column are the L2, L3 and L4 labels. In the second column you'll find the bone density values for each vertebra that was measured. Other columns indicate additional measurements known as the T-score and Z-score. Their meanings are explained later in the chapter. The numbers on the bottom row are an average for the three vertebrae combined.

The colored graph that accompanies the summary table compares the average bone density for the three lumbar vertebrae measured with the normal bone density readings for an individual of the same age. The blue area crossing the graph represents the normal range.

The black square positioned on the graph indicates that the person being tested is in his or her early 40s with a bone density of around 1.27. (The table shows the value as exactly 1.272.) This

Region	Bone density	Young-adult T-score	Age-matched Z-score
L2	1.270	0.6	1.1
L3	1.243	0.4	0.9
L4	1.301	0.8	1.3
L2-L4	1.272	0.6	1.1

Spine L2-L4

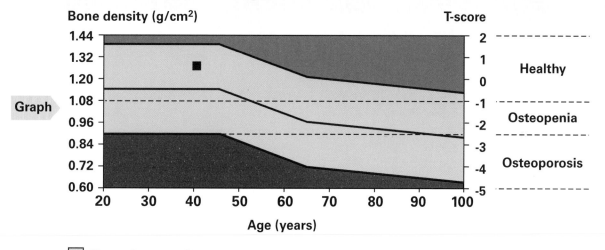

Graph

Normal range of bone density for lumbar vertebrae over time

person has excellent bone density in the lumbar region, with a score in the upper half of the range for individuals around age 40.

Bone density test results from other skeletal locations will include similar images, tables and graphs. On the next two pages are the results of a bone density test performed on the left hip. The black square on the top colored graph indicates that the person who had the test was about 40-years-old,

and that he or she has normal bone density of the hip for his or her age.

White lines superimposed on the accompanying image indicate four regions where bone density was measured (see page 85). They are the femoral neck, shaft, trochanter and Ward's triangle (which is actually a square on the image). The summary table at the very top of page 84 lists each region individually and provides an average score (total) of the four regions.

Region	Bone density	Young-adult T-score	Age-matched Z-score
Neck	0.919	-0.5	0.0
Ward	0.734	-1.4	-0.8
Troch	0.724	-0.6	-0.2
Shaft	1.118	-	-
Total	0.932	-0.6	-0.1

Summary table

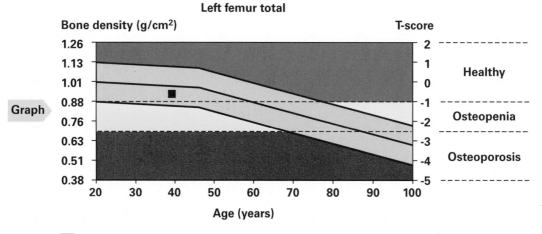

Left femur total

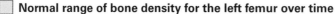

☐ Normal range of bone density for the left femur over time

Graph

Spine L2-L4

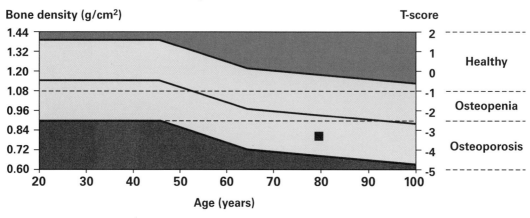

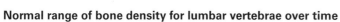

☐ Normal range of bone density for lumbar vertebrae over time

Results reveal osteoporosis The bottom graph shows the results of bone density test of the spine in someone around 80 years old. This person would be diagnosed as having osteoporosis.

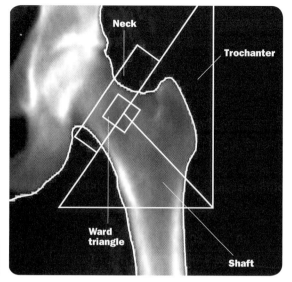

Neck

Trochanter

Ward triangle

Shaft

© MFMER

DXA image A DXA test of the hip has the same elements as a bone density test of the spine: an image, summary table and graph. The four regions of the hip measured in this test are indicated by the white outlines. Test results indicate someone in his or her early 40s with good bone density of the left hip (femur).

What do the results look like when someone has osteoporosis? Look at the bottom graph on the opposite page. This test was performed on the lumbar region of the spine. The location of the black square indicates that this person is around 80 years old, and it shows that the person's bone density score is approximately 0.75. That score is in the low range for an individual this age. You can see that the black square falls below the separation line (bottom dashed line) between osteopenia and

osteoporosis. Therefore, this person would be diagnosed with osteoporosis.

What hasn't been explained so far from the examples presented are what's known as the T-score and Z-score. Both scores provide important information to your doctor. The T-score figures prominently into any diagnosis of osteoporosis. Z-scores, meanwhile, are used to help identify osteoporosis in premenopausal women and men younger than age 50.

Due to differences in the machines used to measure bone density (densitometers), there's variation in how these numbers are derived. The sections that follow will help you understand what the scores mean and how they're used.

Understanding T-scores

Your T-score represents your bone density compared with normal bone density in a healthy, young adult of the same sex. On the test report, the difference between the two is displayed in standard deviations (SD) above or below the mean value. Think of the mean value as the average.

You may wonder why your bone density is compared to that of an individual who's considerably younger than you? There's actually a good reason for doing it this way. It allows everyone to be compared to the same common baseline — in other words, to begin at the same starting point. No one expects a 60-year-old woman to have the same T-score as a woman who is 30 years old. The value comes in knowing the difference — how much your bone density varies from normal.

The T-score you receive on a bone density test expresses how much you differ (deviate) from the average (mean value). If your T-score is 0.0, you don't deviate at all because you match the mean of the group you're being compared with. If your T-score is -1.0, your bone density is lower than average by one standard deviation. Likewise, if your T-score is +0.5, your bone density is higher than average by one-half of a standard deviation.

When reviewing your T-score to determine if you may have low bone density (osteopenia) or osteoporosis, your doctor will likely follow the official guidelines of the World Health Organization (WHO) and the National Osteoporosis Foundation. According to these guidelines:

- If your T-score is within one standard deviation of the average, that is, between +1.0 and -1.0, you have normal bone density.
- If your T-score is -1.0 to -2.4, you have low bone density, what's called osteopenia.
- If your T-score is -2.5 or lower, you have osteoporosis.
- If your T-score is -2.5 or lower and you've broken one or more bones, you have severe osteoporosis.

These same criteria apply to both men and women. For most bone density tests, a -1.0 standard deviation equals a 10 to 12 percent decrease in bone density. Therefore, a T-score of -2.5 would mean your bone density is about 25 to 30 percent lower than that of an average healthy woman or man at peak bone mass.

T-scores from different bones in your skeleton can't be compared. Generally, when more than one bone is tested, doctors use the lowest T-score to diagnose osteoporosis. For example, if you have a T-score of -2.7 in your spine and -2.0 in your hip, the spine T-score would be used to indicate osteoporosis.

Test results may be a good indicator of osteoporosis, but they're not a complete diagnosis. Being told that you have os-

Region	Bone density	Young-adult T-score	Age-matched Z-score
L2	1.270	0.6	1.1
L3	1.243	0.4	0.9
L4	1.301	0.8	1.3
L2-L4	1.272	0.6	1.1

T-score referred to for diagnosis

Interpreting the scores The third and fourth columns on this table indicate the T-scores and Z-scores for the three vertebrae measured in this test. The bottom T-score — the average score of all three vertebrae — is the one a doctor would consider most heavily for a diagnosis of osteoporosis. A T-score of +0.6 is higher than average by 0.6 of a standard deviation.

teopenia (a T-score in the range of -1.0 to -2.4) doesn't guarantee that you'll develop osteoporosis, but it does mean that you want to avoid further loss of bone mass.

Understanding Z-scores

Your Z-score is the number of standard deviations above or below what's expected not only for someone of your sex, but also for someone of your age, weight and ethnic origin.

While your Z-score is a good indicator of how normal or abnormal your bone density is for your age, it's not used to determine if you have osteoporosis, unless you're a premenopausal woman, a male younger than age 50 or a child. In these groups, the Z-score is useful because it can point to a secondary form of osteoporosis — something other than aging or menopause, the most common causes of osteoporosis, that may be contributing to bone loss.

A Z-score lower than -2.0 suggests that secondary osteoporosis may be responsible for bone loss. A doctor will likely try to determine if an underlying disease or condition may be responsible. If a cause can be identified, the disease or condition can often be treated and bone loss slowed or stopped.

In general, the lower your Z-score, the more likely something other than aging or menopause is contributing to your bone loss. However, fewer than 3 percent of adults have a Z-score lower than -2.0. And fewer than 1 percent have a Z-score lower than -3.0.

It's possible to have a normal Z-score and an abnormal T-score. In fact, this is quite common among older adults. The reason is because most everyone experiences a decline in bone density with age. By the time many people reach their 80s, their bone density may be normal for people their age, according to their Z-score, but they may have osteopenia or osteoporosis, according to their T-score.

If you're a bit confused by these two scores, don't worry. Your doctor or a member of the medical staff will help explain the numbers and answer your questions.

How are the numbers used?

The T-scores and Z-scores are important pieces of information when determining if you have, or may be at risk of, osteoporosis. Let's look at two imaginary examples that illustrate how the numbers are used to assess bone health and diagnose osteoporosis.

Example 1

Sally is 59 years old. She has completed menopause. She doesn't smoke and doesn't drink alcohol in excess. She doesn't take corticosteroids and she's never broken a bone. However, her mother had osteoporosis. Concerned about her own chances of getting the disease, Sally talks to her doctor. Given her age and her family history, her doctor arranges for Sally to have a bone density test of her hip using dual energy X-ray absorptiometry (DXA).

Following the test, Sally studies the printout of her test results (see the graph on the opposite page). She notices how normal bone density for the left femur gradually declines with age, and the decline becomes more pronounced around age 45. A black square on the graph indicates that Sally's T-score is -2.3. That means that her bone density is 2.3 standard deviations below the mean value of that of a group of healthy, young women.

Although she doesn't have osteoporosis — which generally requires a T-score of -2.5 or lower — Sally is told that she

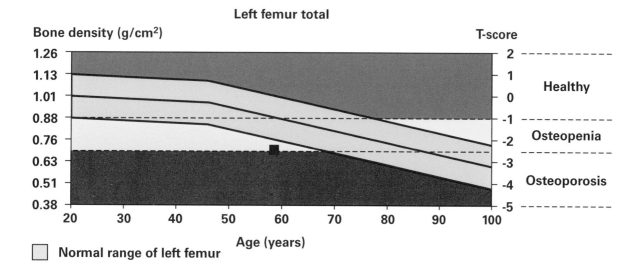

Left femur total

Bone density (g/cm²) ... T-score

Healthy

Osteopenia

Osteoporosis

Age (years)

☐ **Normal range of left femur**

has osteopenia and that she's at risk of osteoporosis if she experiences more bone loss in the future.

Sally's Z-score, meanwhile, is -0.7, seven-tenths of a standard deviation below the norm for a woman of her age and race. Her Z-score isn't low enough to suggest that her bone loss is due to a secondary cause, such as an underlying disease or disorder or a particular medication.

Example 2

Kristen is 42 years old. Seven years ago, she had her uterus and ovaries surgically removed (a total hysterectomy). She wasn't given estrogen after surgery. She doesn't smoke or drink alcohol in

excess. She has no family history of osteoporosis and she's never broken a bone.

Kristen's T-score is the same as Sally's: -2.3 (see the graph on page 90). But Kristen is 15 years younger than Sally, which gives her an additional 15 years to lose more bone mass. For this reason, she's at greater risk of developing osteoporosis.

Kristen's Z-score is -2.3, the same as her T-score. A Z-score that low typically suggests that something in addition to natural aging is affecting her bone density. In Kristen's case, menopause caused by her hysterectomy and the drop in her estrogen level that followed may have triggered a sudden and early loss of bone mass.

Left femur total

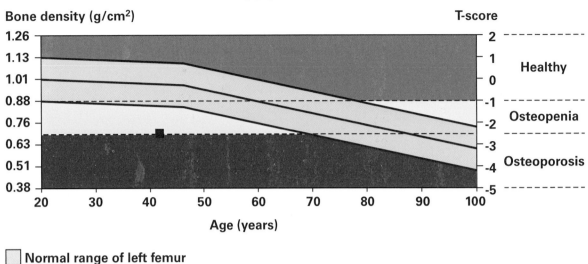

Normal range of left femur

These two examples illustrate how similar bone density scores can have a different meaning for different people. You may have the same T-score as your neighbor, but one of you may develop osteoporosis and the other may not. Although Kristen doesn't have osteoporosis, she's at much greater risk of getting it than is Sally because she's younger and has more time to lose bone.

Other risk factors

T-scores and Z-scores are both statistical probabilities based on groups of people with similar characteristics. However, you are a unique individual with a specific genetic makeup and life-style, which also affect risk. That's why when your doctor considers your risk of bone fracture, he or she takes into account additional factors:

Age

The older you are, the more likely you are to get osteoporosis and break a bone because of it. Daily wear and tear over time causes your bones to become more fragile and less able to absorb shock.

Your sex

Approximately 80 percent of individuals in the U.S. with osteoporosis are

Predicting your 10-year fracture risk

After you've completed a bone mineral density test, your doctor will combine the results with additional information gathered during your health history and physical exam to get an accurate picture of your fracture risk.

Your test results — mainly your T-score at the femoral neck — and other information about you are entered into a fracture risk assessment tool developed by the World Health Organization (WHO) called FRAX. FRAX is used in people with reduced bone density (osteopenia) to determine who should receive treatment. The tool analyzes the information provided to calculate your probability of a fracture within the next 10 years.

A bone mineral density test is the standard for diagnosing osteoporosis, but the test results don't take into account other factors that are important to properly evaluate fracture risk. These include ethnicity, body mass index, prior fractures, family fracture history, medication use, chronic illnesses, tobacco use and alcohol consumption. The geographic area in which you live also is considered in the fracture risk assessment. Fracture probability varies markedly among different regions of the world. Countries with the highest risk include Norway, Iceland, Sweden, Denmark and the United States. Those with the lowest risk are Turkey, Korea, Venezuela and Chile.

FRAX was developed to help doctors better identify and treat women and men at high risk of a debilitating bone fracture. With this tool, doctors can identify individuals who wouldn't have been candidates for treatment based solely on bone density test results.

While FRAX is helpful for predicting fractures, it cannot indicate which treatment will work best to reduce your fracture risk. Your doctor will consider a variety of factors in devising a treatment plan.

women. Women are three times as likely as men to break a bone due to osteoporosis.

Body frame

Men and women who have small body frames generally have a higher risk of osteoporosis and subsequent bone fracture because they tend to have less bone mass to draw from as they age. For larger women and men with a thick-boned frame, the risk is less.

Previous fracture

If you've already broken a bone as an adult, you're at increased risk of breaking another one, even if you don't have osteoporosis. This is true for both women and men.

Family history of hip fracture

If a parent — either a mother or father — experienced a fractured hip, your risk of hip fracture is increased.

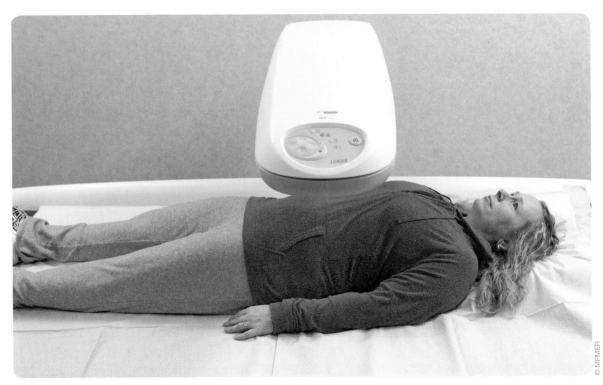

© MFMER

Determining risk Bone density test results aren't the only factor considered when determining an individual's risk of osteoporosis and bone fracture. Lifestyle and personal health factors also are important.

Smoking

Individuals who smoke are more likely to experience osteoporosis and bone fractures. That's because smoking interferes with the production of the hormones estrogen and testosterone. Smoking also disrupts calcium absorption and the bone formation part of the remodeling cycle.

Alcohol

Excessive use of alcohol over a long period of time is damaging to bone because alcohol is toxic to bone-building osteoblasts. Chronic heavy drinking also lowers levels of the hormones estrogen and testosterone.

Use of glucocorticoids

These medications are especially hard on your bones. They lower bone mass by slowing bone formation, they temporarily speed bone resorption, and they decrease levels of estrogen and testosterone. Risk of osteoporosis and subsequent fracture is greatest in individuals who take oral or intravenous glucocorticoids for more than three to six months. Risk is reduced with inhaled glucocorticoids.

Rheumatoid arthritis

Studies suggest that having rheumatoid arthritis increases your risk of osteoporosis and fracture. Joint damage and limited mobility that accompany rheumatoid arthritis increase fracture risk. Some medications used to treat the disease also can damage bone and put you at higher risk of osteoporosis.

Other causes of osteoporosis

Secondary osteoporosis refers to certain diseases, surgical procedures or drugs that can accelerate bone loss and increase your chances of a fracture. Other medical conditions that can affect osteoporosis risk include excess production of thyroid hormones (hyperthyroidism), excess production of parathyroid hormones (hyerparathyroidism), type 1 and type 2 diabetes, and liver disease. Long-term use of certain medications also may play a role (see page 182).

When your doctor is determining your fracture risk, he or she will take into account medical conditions and medications that may increase your odds of breaking a bone. For more information on secondary causes of osteoporosis, see Chapter 12.

In summary

Bone density tests are important, but keep in mind that they aren't the be-all and end-all to determining your bone health. There's more to diagnosing osteoporosis and fracture risk than a number from a densitometer. Before jumping to conclusions, discuss your bone density test results with a doctor. It's important that he or she connect all of the dots to create a complete picture of your bone health.

Part 2

Prevention
and treatment

Chapter 7

Developing an action plan

It's never too early to fight back against osteoporosis or too late to stop the condition in its tracks. Whether you're trying to prevent osteoporosis or you need to treat it, the goal is the same: You want to maintain your bone health to ensure a low risk of fracture. And regardless if prevention or treatment is your aim, the steps you'll take to protect your bones are the same.

Understanding your role in the prevention or treatment of osteoporosis is vital for success. That's because many of the steps require your active participation. Working together, you and your doctor will want to develop an action plan that includes key strategies related to diet, exercise and medications. Think of your action plan as your "how-to" blueprint for keeping your bones healthy.

Even if you don't have osteoporosis, an action plan is still important. A good plan can greatly reduce your risk of getting the disease. Ideally, prevention begins in childhood and it continues throughout life. The more you build up your bones during your early years, the less likely you are to develop osteoporosis later in life.

Strong bones for a lifetime

A successful action plan involves several elements that contribute to overall bone health. These elements include good nutrition — including an adequate intake of calcium and vitamin D — regular physical activity, healthy habits and behaviors, good posture, and careful use of medications.

When combined, these elements support and strengthen one another to help you prevent or manage osteoporosis, keep you healthy, and maintain your overall quality of life. Each element is discussed in this chapter to show why the element is essential to your action plan and how it interrelates to other elements of your plan. Future chapters discuss specific elements in more detail, providing additional information and demonstrating how strategies related to it can be put to practical use.

In establishing an action plan, consider these objectives:

- Maximize the development of your skeleton. As a child or young adult, the focus is on attaining a high peak bone mass. As an older adult, the goal is to stabilize existing bone mass.
- Prevent fractures. Bones weakened by the depletion of calcium and other minerals are more likely to break.
- Relieve the symptoms of fractures, stooped posture and chronic pain, should they occur.
- Improve your balance and the ability to move and be active.

Success in meeting these objectives depends in part on your commitment to your action plan. It's up to you to stick with daily routines and be willing to change some of your behaviors.

At the same time, you don't have to do it alone. As with any chronic disease, it's important to maintain good relationships with professionals, as well as with family and friends. Several kinds of doctors can help treat or prevent osteoporosis, including endocrinologists, rheumatologists, general practitioners, internists, gynecologists, rehabilitation specialists and orthopedists.

Often your own doctor is the best person to work with because he or she knows you personally, including your medical history. In dealing with certain parts of your action plan, you may also find it useful to consult a dietitian, or a physical or occupational therapist.

Diet and nutrition

Good bone health starts with good nutrition. To keep your bones healthy, you need a balanced diet that includes enough calcium, vitamin D and other nutrients that your body requires to perform its daily functions. Calcium

Starting young

The secret to preventing osteoporosis is to make your skeleton as strong as it can be by doing everything you can to help it reach its peak bone mass. (For more discussion of peak bone mass, see Chapter 2.) By eating right and staying physically active during the years when bone mass is increasing — from childhood to approximately age 30 — you can lessen the impact of bone loss that occurs naturally in your later years.

Parents and grandparents can help children develop habits that will benefit their bones for the rest of their lives. Start by making sure children get enough calcium. Young people often have diets deficient in calcium. Good overall nutrition also is important. Some young women diet excessively in a quest to be thin and deprive themselves of valuable nutrients. Low body weight puts bones at risk. Conversely, studies show that young women can increase their bone mass by increasing calcium intake in their diet.

Many children love soft drinks, which have no calcium content. Parents can do their kids a favor by skipping the soda and offering milk or calcium-fortified juice instead. Milk and fruit juice are among the top sources of vitamins, calcium and magnesium for children in the United States.

Parents and grandparents can also encourage physical activity as part of the family routine, whether it's an evening walk after dinner, swimming, bowling, a canoe trip, or a game of basketball or tennis. Regular physical activity is essential for building strong muscles and bones.

and vitamin D are essential nutrients for maximizing and preserving bone mass.

Getting adequate calcium and vitamin D can reduce the risk of hip and nonvertebral fractures in older adults. Protein and other nutrients, such as the minerals phosphorus, sodium and magnesium, also play important roles in keeping your bones strong.

Calcium: The foundation

Calcium is found in every cell in your body, although about 99 percent of it lies in your bones and teeth. Because calcium is a major component of bone, you need adequate amounts of the mineral throughout your life to achieve and maintain peak bone mass.

Calcium is also needed for your heart, muscles and nerves to function properly and for your blood to clot normally. It's important your bloodstream always contain an adequate supply of calcium. Fortunately, the body has built-in safeguards to regulate the level of calcium in your blood — allowing for neither too little nor too much.

Each day, you lose some calcium from your body. It's excreted by way of urine and feces and, to a lesser extent, sweat. This continual loss of calcium means that your body requires constant replenishment.

If you don't consume enough of the mineral in your diet, your parathyroid glands will release parathyroid hormone, which in turn stimulates your bones to release calcium. Your bones give up calcium in order to keep the calcium level in your blood normal. If this action occurs repeatedly over a long period of time, your bones continue to lose calcium and your bone density level decreases.

Calcium requirements

Calcium is essential during childhood and adolescence when your skeleton is growing rapidly. And contrary to popular belief, your need for dietary calcium increases — not decreases — with age.

This is because as you get older, your body becomes less efficient at absorbing calcium and vitamin D from the foods you eat and at retaining calcium in your kidneys. For women, a drop in estrogen levels at menopause further reduces calcium absorption. In addition, older adults are more likely to have chronic medical problems and use medications that may impair calcium

Recommended daily calcium for adults

Age	Adequate intake (milligrams/day)	Upper limit (milligrams/day)
Men		
19-50 years	1,000	2,500
51-70 years	1,000	2,000
71+ years	1,200	2,000
Women		
19-50 years	1,000	2,500
51+ years	1,200	2,000

Note that the upper limit represents the safe boundary — it's not how much you should aim to get. If you exceed the upper limit, you may increase your risk of health problems related to excessive calcium.

Institute of Medicine, 2010

absorption. All of these changes put greater pressure on your body to maintain sufficient calcium levels in your bloodstream.

Unfortunately, many people don't get the calcium they need. It's recommended that adults get 1,000 to 1,200 milligrams (mg) of calcium a day to keep their bones strong. The typical American diet provides less — about 600 mg — well below recommended adult levels.

Groups most likely to consume too little calcium are boys and girls ages 9 to 13, girls ages 14 to 18, women between the ages of 51 and 70, and both men and women older than age 70.

Researchers cite several possible reasons for the calcium deficiency. Foremost is the fact that people are eating fewer dairy products. Soda, bottled water and sports drinks are often substituted for milk, which is high in calcium. Some people also avoid milk because of intolerance to the sugar in milk (lactose). Or they believe that milk leads to weight gain or conditions such as acne. In addition, people aren't eating enough fruits and vegetables, which also contain vitamins and minerals important to bone health.

During pregnancy and lactation

During pregnancy, a mother's body needs extra calcium for the developing fetus. To get additional calcium, the mother's ability to absorb the mineral from the intestines is increased — a nifty trick of Mother Nature. During lactation a mother's kidneys conserve calcium, making more of the mineral available for her and the baby.

Because of these changes in the body, the recommended calcium intake for women during pregnancy and lactation is the same as that for all women of the same age. Nevertheless, if you're pregnant, talk to your doctor about meeting calcium requirements.

One way to increase the calcium in your diet is to know which foods are rich in calcium and include them in your meals. An easy way to get adequate calcium is to have a glass of milk with every meal. Another way is to take a calcium supplement. These topics, as well as an overview of good nutrition, are discussed in Chapter 8.

Don't overdo calcium supplements

While it's important that you have adequate calcium in your diet, it's also important how you get that calcium — and that you don't get too much. A couple of recent studies suggested that men and women who take calcium supplements may be at increased risk of heart attacks compared with those who don't take supplements. However, the number of actual heart attacks among those in the studies was small.

In comparison, the researchers didn't find any link between dietary calcium — the calcium in food and beverages — and heart attack risk. In fact, the higher the calcium intake, the less risk of heart attack.

More research is needed before doctors know the effect calcium supplements may have on heart attack risk. As with any health issue, it's important to talk to your doctor to determine what's best in your particular situation.

Vitamin D: Unlocking the door for calcium

The amount of calcium you consume is not the sole answer to building strong bones. Your body must maintain a balance between how much calcium is absorbed from the food you eat and how much is eliminated from your body.

Calcium absorption takes place as your intestines extract the mineral from the food you eat and move it into your bloodstream. Calcium excretion occurs primarily through urine, feces and sweat. Poor absorption and increased excretion can upset the calcium balance and weaken your bones.

Enter vitamin D. Vitamin D is as critical to your bone health as is calcium. It plays an important role in maintaining the absorption-excretion balance by increasing calcium absorption in the small intestine. Think of vitamin D as the key that unlocks a door, allowing calcium to leave the intestines and enter the bloodstream. If you don't get enough vitamin D, the level of calcium circulating in your bloodstream drops.

When calcium levels in your blood become too low, your parathyroid hormone signals your bones to release more calcium into circulation. This isn't

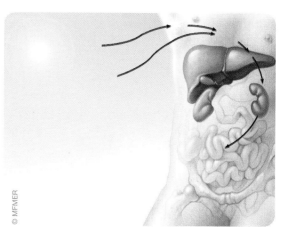

How your body makes vitamin D When you're exposed to sunlight, the sun's ultraviolet rays change a chemical in your skin to an inactive form of vitamin D. Inactive vitamin D is also contained in some foods. Your liver and kidneys make two more chemical changes to vitamin D that activate the nutrient. In its active form, vitamin D helps absorb calcium for maintaining healthy bones.

good because it reduces the amount of calcium in your bones. Continually robbing your bones of calcium can cause them to weaken. This is why it's important that you get enough vitamin D in addition to enough calcium.

Sources of vitamin D
The main source of vitamin D for most people is sunlight. Ultraviolet (UV) radiation from the sun stimulates your skin to synthesize vitamin D. As much as 90 percent of your vitamin D supply can come from sunlight.

Recommended daily intake of vitamin D

Age	Recommended intake (international units/day)	Upper limit (international units/day)
1-3 years	600	2,500
4-8 years	600	3,000
9-70 years	600	4,000
71+ years	800	4,000

Note that the upper limit represents the safe boundary — it's not how much you should aim to get.

Institute of Medicine, 2010

How much vitamin D you convert from sunlight depends on many factors, including the season; the latitude at which you live; the amount of sunshine and air pollution in your region; your age; the condition of your skin, liver and kidneys; and the type of clothing you wear.

Using sunscreen and spending long periods of time indoors, especially in the winter months, prevent some people from getting adequate vitamin D. In addition, in some northern latitudes, solar radiation isn't strong enough in the winter to produce adequate vitamin D in skin. In these situations, when the body doesn't get enough vitamin D from the sun, it depends on its stored supply of the vitamin or dietary sources of vitamin D.

Only a few foods are naturally rich in vitamin D. They include fatty fish, fish liver oils (including cod liver oil), liver and egg yolks. The milk you buy at the grocery store is usually fortified with vitamin D.

Vitamin D requirements

Getting enough vitamin D is necessary at any age. Most infants and children in the United States get enough vitamin D because it's added to milk. Although consumption of milk often decreases during adolescence, vitamin D deficiency is unusual in this age group. It's more common in older adults, and there are a number of reasons why.

- Older adults don't always consume enough foods and beverages fortified with vitamin D, such as milk.

- Your ability to absorb vitamin D from what you eat and drink tends to diminish with age.
- Many older adults spend less time in the sun, particularly in northern latitudes during the winter months.
- With age, your skin becomes less able to synthesize vitamin D, and organs such as the kidneys and liver may become less efficient at processing it.

To help ensure an adequate amount of vitamin D from sunlight, some experts recommend getting 10 to 15 minutes of midday sun exposure on your face, arms and hands at least twice a week. This recommendation is dependent on individual skin sensitivities.

When you're exposed to the sun's rays, remember many factors can reduce the effectiveness of sunlight for producing vitamin D. These include sunscreen, light filtered through a window, air pollution and the weakness of solar radiation in winter. If you're affected by any of these factors, you may benefit from vitamin D supplements. Individuals who take steroid medications such as prednisone or hydrocortisone may require additional vitamin D.

Body weight and osteoporosis

Most of us have heard about the dangers of being overweight. Among other things, obesity can put you at increased risk of a heart attack and stroke. But being too thin isn't healthy either, especially when it comes to your bones. Your diet should include enough calories to maintain a normal body weight. Weight has a powerful effect on bone mass. It increases the load on your skeleton, and your bones compensate by growing stronger.

Women who are very lean run the risk of having low bone mass, excessive bone loss at menopause and increased risk of a fracture. If you're underweight, you want to reach a normal weight — weigh neither too much nor too little. If you're having trouble with your weight or your diet, talk to your doctor or a dietitian.

Other nutrients and your bones

Nutrients other than calcium and vitamin D also can influence your bone health both positively and negatively.

Phosphorus

Phosphorus is important for normal development and maintenance of your bones and tissues. It's present in most foods, including meat, poultry, fish, eggs, dairy products, nuts, legumes, cereals and grains. Phosphate salts are used extensively in processed foods.

Phosphorus consumption in the American diet has risen about 10 to 15 percent in recent decades, due primarily to increased use of food additives and consumption of carbonated beverages. There's speculation that an excess of phosphorus may have adverse effects on your skeleton, possibly increasing the risk of low bone density.

Sodium

Sodium chloride, the main component in table salt, increases calcium excretion through urine. Although uncommon, a diet that's high in sodium may adversely affect the calcium balance in your bloodstream. Most American adults consume more than the recommended limit of 2,300 milligrams of sodium daily.

Protein

Protein is one of the building blocks of bone and it's essential to build and repair tissue. It also aids in fracture healing and is necessary for the body's immune system to function properly. Most Americans consume more than

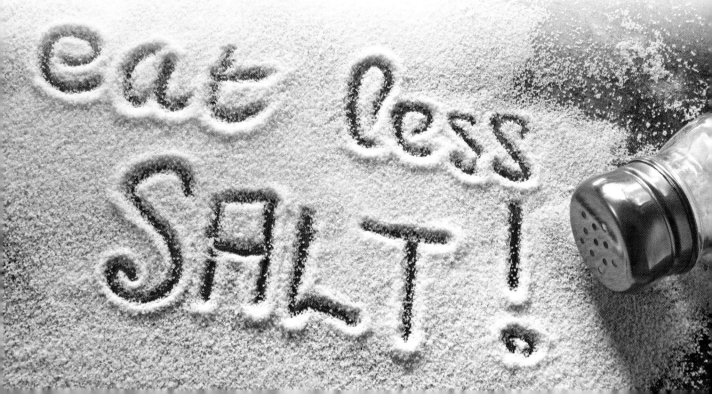

the recommended amount of daily protein, which is 46 grams for women and 56 grams for men. For reference, 16 grams of protein is found in 2 cups of milk, and 3 ounces of meat contains about 21 grams of protein.

Studies suggest that a high-protein diet may increase the amount of calcium excreted through your kidneys. On the other hand, a low-protein diet may interfere with calcium absorption in the intestines. A diet containing a moderate level of protein is likely best.

The bottom line? It's best to eat a balanced diet that includes the recommended amounts of calcium, phosphorus, sodium and protein. Too much or too little of these nutrients isn't good for your health, or your bones. See Chapter 8 for more information about nutrition.

Physical activity

Physical activity on a regular basis is another key component of any action plan to prevent or treat osteoporosis. Studies show that regular exercise early in life helps you achieve a higher peak bone mass. During your adult years, exercise can help slow bone loss, maintain your posture and strengthen your

cardiovascular health. Exercise also improves your balance, coordination and muscle strength, all of which reduce the risk of falling and breaking a bone. Evidence also indicates that physical activity improves muscle function.

Activity builds bone

Bone is living tissue that can strengthen — or weaken — in relation to how much it's used. The greater the demands you place on bone, the stronger and denser it becomes.

When you perform an action such as hitting a tennis ball or landing on your feet after a jump, chemical messengers instruct your arm bones or leg bones to be ready to handle that impact again. Repeating the action over time reinforces the preparedness of your bones.

If you look closely at X-rays of the arms of a tennis player, you can see that the bones of the dominant arm — the one that holds the racket — are larger and denser than the bones of the other arm. Conversely, people who are put on bed rest or otherwise immobilized lose bone strength quickly due to lack of activity.

Every bit of activity helps. Being active includes all of the motions of daily living. Moving around throughout the day is good for you. Better yet is more structured activity. This may include taking a walk or playing a round of golf. Your bones also benefit from resistance exercises, which often involve the use of weights.

If you have osteoporosis or may be at risk, before starting an exercise program talk with your doctor about what types of activities are appropriate for you. Certain exercises you may want to avoid or limit. Physical activity is discussed in more detail in Chapter 9.

Perfecting your posture

In addition to activities that strengthen your bones, you also want to include those that help strengthen your back muscles and improve your posture. Good posture is crucial to preventing falls and avoiding an excessively curved back.

Posture refers to the positions of different body parts in relation to one another — whether you're standing, sitting, lying down or moving. Good posture allows your back to follow the mild S-shaped curve of the spine, and it places only minimal strain on your muscles and joints.

Knowing how to sit, stand and move properly can help you avoid fractures and limit the exaggerated curvature of the spine that results from compression fractures. For more on good posture and proper ways to move, see Chapter 11.

Medications

In addition to diet and exercise, medications are often prescribed for people at high risk of developing osteoporosis and those who've been diagnosed with the disease. The main goal of medications is to preserve or increase bone density and prevent fractures.

Most prescription medications for osteoporosis are called bone anti-resorptive agents. The term refers to the action of slowing or stopping the breakdown of bone tissue (resorption). By putting the brakes on bone removal, anti-resorptives help bone formation keep pace. This often allows bone density to increase over time.

Medications that promote the formation of new bone tissue also may be prescribed. They're most commonly used to treat women and men with severe forms of osteoporosis, including those at a high risk of fracture and who

Complementary and alternative treatments

To date, no specific complementary or alternative treatment has been proved effective specifically for treating osteoporosis. Getting adequate calcium and vitamin D is the cornerstone of osteoporosis prevention and treatment. Calcium and vitamin D are the only two supplements that have been consistently shown to decrease fracture rates. Dietary sources are preferable, but many people may need a calcium and vitamin D supplement, especially if they don't get sufficient high-calcium foods and exposure to the sun.

Soy isoflavones or ipriflavone also may help prevent bone loss. Ipriflavone is a semisynthetic organic compound manufactured from the isoflavone daidzein. In combination with adequate calcium and vitamin D, soy isoflavones and ipriflavone may help increase bone mineral density. Many herbs also are promoted for osteoporosis, but there's not enough good clinical evidence to support their use.

Another alternative practice that may be beneficial is tai chi. Research suggests it may be a safe alternative to conventional exercise among postmenopausal women for maintaining bone mineral density. Tai chi is a mind-body practice that originated in China as a martial art. It consists of slow and gentle body moves, while breathing deeply and meditating. Tai chi is sometimes called "moving meditation." The benefits of tai chi appeared similar to those of conventional exercise. However, tai chi may also improve balance to help reduce the risk of falls.

For individuals with osteoporosis who have experienced one or more osteoporotic fractures of the spine, studies suggest that treatments such as biofeedback, meditation and relaxation techniques may be useful in treating chronic pain, which can accompany such fractures. Various methods for managing chronic pain are discussed in Chapter 14.

If you have osteoporosis, be cautious about two forms of alternative and complementary medicine that could worsen your condition — chiropractic treatment and massage. These therapies aren't recommended because they can cause or aggravate spinal fractures. Before trying any form of spinal manipulation, it's best to talk with your doctor.

If you're considering any complementary or alternative therapy, gather as much information about the treatment as you can. Bring the information with you to your next appointment and seek out your doctor's advice.

haven't responded well to other forms of treatment.

For more detailed information about medications, including those under investigation, see Chapter 10.

Healthy behaviors

Along with a balanced diet, physical activity and medications, you may need to direct your attention to other aspects of your life that are harming your bones. For example, stopping smoking and avoiding excessive use of alcohol are important steps in treating or preventing osteoporosis.

Avoid smoking

Studies show that smoking increases the rate of bone loss. Women who smoke have lower estrogen levels than do women who don't smoke. Women smokers also tend to undergo menopause earlier, and cigarette smokers tend to be thinner. All of these factors increase the risk of osteoporosis and possible fractures.

Avoid excessive alcohol use

Studies indicate that consuming more than a moderate amount of alcohol — defined as no more than two drinks a day for men age 65 and younger and one drink a day for women and men older than 65 — can hasten bone loss and reduce your body's ability to absorb calcium. Alcohol can affect hormones that regulate calcium levels and reduce the formation of new bone. People who drink heavily also are more prone to fractures because of an increased risk of falling.

Meeting the challenge

All of the elements described in this chapter, including diet, physical activity, correct posture, medications and healthy behaviors, can help you maintain bone strength and avoid fractures. Each element helps to address a vital aspect of your health. However, no individual element is sufficient in itself to prevent or treat osteoporosis — each component works best in combination with the others.

The chapters that follow provide practical suggestions for implementing your action plan. By being proactive and involved in your health, you can enjoy a more active, fulfilling life.

Chapter 8

Eating for healthy bones

Like any living tissue, bones need nutrients so that they can grow and maintain themselves. Most nutrients aren't produced by the body; they must be provided by food. A lack of nutrients in your diet can lead to stunted growth, weaker bones and other medical conditions. In other words, the better your diet, the better your health. And the stronger your bones, the less chance you have of developing osteoporosis.

Calcium and vitamin D have received the most attention for their roles in preventing and treating osteoporosis. But other nutrients also play a supporting role in ensuring bone health. They include the minerals magnesium, potassium and fluoride; vitamins C, K and A; and disease-fighting plant compounds called phytochemicals. There's also evidence that watching your calorie intake and maintaining a healthy weight may prevent or reduce your risk of osteoporosis.

The previous chapter talked about diet in the context of how to develop an action plan for preventing or treating osteoporosis. This chapter discusses the basics of good nutrition as well as practical ways to ensure that your diet maximizes bone health.

Good nutrition in a nutshell

Variety isn't just the spice of life, it's the basis for a healthy diet. No single food provides all of the nutrients your body needs. Eating a variety of foods ensures you'll get the nutrients you need to achieve a healthy weight, enjoy good health and maintain strong bones.

A simple approach for achieving and maintaining a healthy diet is to follow basic nutrition guidelines. Nutrition guidelines promote variety, balance and moderation in your food choices. Key recommendations for a healthy diet are often summarized as follows:

- Eat more vegetables, fruits and whole grains.
- Limit protein and fat.
- Choose foods that are good sources of calcium.
- Limit sugar, salt and phosphate additives.
- Limit consumption of alcohol and caffeine.

Eat more vegetables, fruits and whole grains

Studies show that eating more vegetables and fruits — and less protein from meat sources — leads to improved bone health. Choose a variety of vegetables, fruits and whole grains for your daily meals. These foods are generally lower in calories and fat, so you don't have to worry as much about how much of the food you eat. Fruits

and vegetables are also high in fiber, essential vitamins and minerals, and phytochemicals, substances that may help protect against a variety of diseases, including osteoporosis.

Aim to eat four or more servings of vegetables and three or more servings of fruit each day. It's best to eat fresh foods, not processed foods. Because different fruits and vegetables provide different nutrients, variety is vital. Fruits and vegetables are excellent sources of magnesium, potassium, and vitamins C, K and A. All play a role in maintaining bone health.

Also eat four to eight servings of grains — cereal, bread, rice and pasta — daily. This equals about 6 ounces. You may eat less if you're trying to limit calories. Choose whole grains when possible because they contain more nutrients, especially magnesium and fiber, than do refined grains. You may be eating some whole grains without realizing it, such as oatmeal and popcorn.

Limit protein and fat

For bone health — and good health in general — it's important to eat lean types of protein. The best choices include plant proteins, such as beans and

Nutrients and bone health

Nutrient	Role in bone	Food sources include
Calcium	Major mineral found in bone	See pages 116-117
Vitamin D	Essential for absorbing calcium from food and supplements	Fortified milk and cereals
Potassium	Adequate amount helps prevent loss of calcium in urine	Vegetables, fruits, legumes and milk
Vitamin K	Involved in bone formation	Dark green leafy vegetables, fruits and some vegetable oils
Vitamin C	Inadequate consumption associated with low bone density	Citrus fruit and juices, peppers, broccoli, tomatoes, and green leafy vegetables
Vitamin A	Essential for bone remodeling (natural "recycling" of bone)	Darkly colored (orange or red) fruits and vegetables
Magnesium	Adequate intake is associated with higher bone density	Legumes, vegetables, nuts, seeds, fruit, grain, fish and dairy
Phosphorus	Balance needed; consuming too much phosphorus and too little calcium may stimulate the body to reduce bone mass.	Go easy on foods and beverages higher in phosphorus with little calcium, including carbonated cola beverages and processed foods such as chips, breaded items and instant sauces.
Sodium	Causes loss of calcium in urine; more calcium needed to offset loss	Processed foods such as cured meats, pickled items, canned salted soups, canned vegetables, fast foods, chips and more

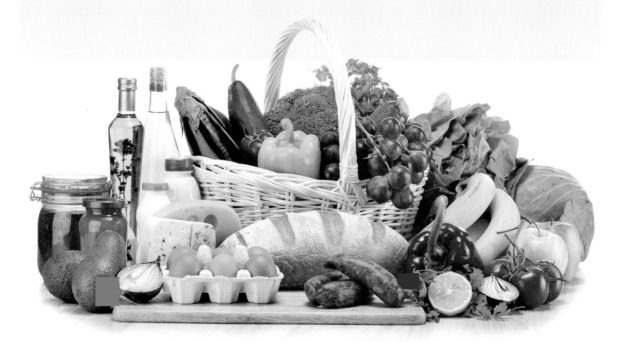

nuts, as well as fish, skinless poultry and lean cuts of meat. Plant proteins are rich in vitamins, minerals and estrogen-like plant compounds that help preserve bone.

Try to limit the total amount of protein from all sources to 5 to 6 ounces daily. A diet too high or too low in protein is associated with bone loss. In addition, if you eat too much protein, you may be less likely to eat healthier fruits, vegetables and whole grains.

As for fat, you need some of it in your diet in order for your body to function properly. But too much fat or the wrong kind can have a negative impact on your health. Of all foods, fat contains the most calories. This is why health experts recommend eating foods low in fat. The bones of people with a high amount of body fat tend to be stronger than those of people at a normal body weight. However, this isn't a reason to be overweight. There are many other reasons why you want to maintain a healthy weight.

When you do include fat in your diet, the best kinds are monounsaturated fats. These include canola oil, olive oil, and spreads and dressings made from them. Even these fats, however, should be eaten in limited amounts.

Choose good sources of calcium

You know that calcium is a nutrition superstar when it comes to bone health. But if you're like most Americans, you may not be getting enough. The typical American diet provides less than 600 milligrams (mg) of calcium daily, but the recommended daily intake for most adults ranges from 1,000 to 1,200 mg or more. (See Chapter 7 for specific calcium requirements.)

The obvious way to increase your calcium intake is to eat more foods that are high in calcium at your meals. Milk and other dairy products, such as yogurt and cheese, are the richest food sources for calcium. You can choose fat-free and low-fat varieties that contain the same amount of calcium as higher fat products. Milk is also fortified with vitamin D. One serving contains about 125 international units of vitamin D.

Dairy products aren't the only foods rich in calcium. Other sources are listed on pages 116-117. However, it's easier to meet calcium requirements with dairy products than with other foods. For example, 1 cup of milk contains the same amount of calcium as about 4 to 5 cups of broccoli. If you can't or you choose not to eat dairy products,

How much calcium are you getting?

Nondairy calcium-rich foods generally provide about 200 to 300 milligrams (mg) of calcium a day. To calculate your daily calcium intake, assume you get about 250 mg from these nondairy sources. Add 300 mg for each serving of dairy that you consume. A serving generally equates to about 1 cup of milk, 6 ounces of plain yogurt or calcium-fortified juice, or 1½ ounces of hard cheese. Then add the amount of calcium contained in any supplements you take.

Below is an example of a woman whose only dairy serving each day is milk that she has with her cereal. However, because she also takes a calcium supplement, she meets her recommended daily intake:

- Nondairy sources: 250 mg
- Dairy servings (½ cup milk): 150 mg
- One calcium supplement: 600 mg
  Total calcium: 1,000 mg

you may have to work a little harder to make sure you get enough calcium.

If you have difficulty digesting milk, you can meet your calcium needs by consuming lactose-free milk products and calcium-fortified foods or by taking a supplement. (See "Lactose intolerance" on page 126.)

Studies suggest calcium-rich foods are better for you than calcium supplements because foods containing calcium generally include other important

nutrients as well. For example, milk also provides protein, vitamins A, D and B-12, magnesium, riboflavin, potassium, and zinc. Dietary calcium may reduce the risk of high blood pressure and kidney stones, but supplements don't have this effect.

Many foods have calcium added to them — such as breakfast cereals, breads, pasta, rice, pancake and waffle mixes, juices, and soy and almond beverages. Check the labels to determine the nutritional content of these foods.

Food sources of calcium

Foods	Amount	Calories	Calcium (milligrams)
Dairy			
Yogurt, plain, low-fat	1 cup	155	450
Yogurt, with fruit, low-fat	1 cup	225	313
Milk, skim	1 cup	80-100	300
Milk, low-fat (2 percent)	1 cup	120	295
Milk, fat-free, dry powder*	1/3 cup	80	285
Milk, whole	1 cup	150	275
Yogurt, frozen, low-fat	1 cup	150-200	215-295
Pudding, with skim milk	1 cup	240	200
Ice cream (10 percent fat)	1 cup	275	170
Cheese			
Ricotta, part-skim milk	1 cup	340	675
American, processed	1 ounce	105	225
Swiss	1 ounce	105	205
Cheddar	1 ounce	115	205
Mozzarella, part-skim milk	1 ounce	85	205
Cottage, regular from whole milk	1 cup	220	190
Cottage, low-fat (from 1 percent milk)	1 cup	165	140
Cottage, fat-free	1 cup	105	125
Fish and shellfish			
Sardines, canned, with bones	3 ounces	180	325
Salmon, canned, with bones	3 ounces	120	215
Shrimp	3 ounces	85	75
Herring, pickled	3 ounces	225	65
Fruit			
Orange juice, calcium-fortified	1 cup	120	350
Orange	1 medium	65	60
Papaya	1 cup	60	30

*1/3 cup dry milk makes 1 cup fluid milk.
USDA Nutrient Database, release 26, November 2013

Foods	Amount	Calories	Calcium (milligrams)
Vegetables			
Rhubarb (sweetened, cooked or frozen)	1 cup	280	350
Soybeans, green (cooked)	1 cup	255	260
Collard, mustard greens	1 cup	65	270
Spinach (fresh, cooked)	1 cup	40	240
Black-eyed peas, or cow peas	1 cup	160	210
Turnip greens (fresh, cooked)	1 cup	30	200
Chinese cabbage (boiled)	1 cup	20	160
Okra (fresh)	1 cup	35	125
Beans, great northern, white (cooked)	1 cup	210	120
Swiss chard (boiled)	1 cup	35	100
Kale (frozen, cooked)	1 cup	35	95
Broccoli (fresh, cooked)	1 cup	55	60
Carrots (cooked)	1 cup	55	50
Broccoli (raw)	1 cup	30	45
Other foods			
Tofu (soybean curd), calcium-fortified	½ cup	185	860
Almond milk	1 ounce	90	450
Soy milk, calcium-fortified	1 cup	105	300
Tomato soup, with milk	1 cup	140	175
Dark molasses	1 tablespoon	60	170
Pizza with cheese, 24 ounces	1 slice	220	145
Macaroni and cheese, dry mix	1 cup	375	125
Hummus	1 cup	410	95
Sunflower seeds	1 ounce	165	20
Peanuts, roasted	1 ounce	165	15
Cashews, oil-roasted	1 ounce	165	15
Cereal, calcium-fortified	Check label on cereal box		

Bone-healthy meals

Here are two sample menus developed by Mayo Clinic dietitians that provide the recommended amount of daily calcium.

The menus emphasize whole grains, vegetables, fruits and low-fat dairy products. This variety helps provide plentiful amounts of calcium and other nutrients. Each day's menu is based on a diet of 2,000 calories, with no more than 30 percent of the calories coming from fat. Sodium is also limited to 2,300 mg a day or less.

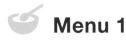 Menu 1

Breakfast
» 1 cup whole-wheat flakes cereal, topped with half a peach
» 2 slices whole-grain toast
» 2 teaspoons soft margarine
» 1 cup skim milk

Lunch
» Turkey sandwich a la Mediterranean:
  1 ounce turkey, 1 ounce part-skim mozzarella cheese, ½ sliced tomato and 1 tablespoon pesto sauce on 2 slices whole-wheat bread
» 1 fresh apple
» 1 cup fresh vegetables: raw baby carrots, celery sticks and broccoli florets
» ¼ cup non-fat cottage cheese (dip)
» 8 ounces cranberry juice

Dinner
» 4 ounces grilled salmon steak
» ½ cup (3 small) roasted new potatoes
» Spinach with feta cheese and almonds (Recipe on page 121)

» 1 whole-wheat roll with margarine
» 1 tablespoon honey
» 1 cup skim milk

Snack (anytime)
» 3 cups air-popped popcorn

Menu 1 nutritional analysis
Food servings
Grain/carbohydrate: 9
Fruits: 4
Vegetables: 4
Protein/dairy: 5
Fats: 4
Sweets: 1

Nutrient content per menu
Calories: 1,950
Fat (g): 51
Saturated fat (g): 14
Cholesterol (mg): 130
Sodium (mg): 2,300
Calcium (mg): 1,150

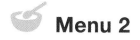

Menu 2

Breakfast
» Omelet: 1 egg, 2 egg whites, 1½ ounces low-fat cheddar cheese, ¼ cup chopped onion and 1¼ cup chopped tomato, 1 teaspoon corn oil
» 1 small cornmeal muffin
» 2 teaspoons fruit spread
» 6 ounces calcium-fortified orange juice
» Decaffeinated coffee with low-fat milk

Lunch
» Wild rice soup (Recipe on page 120)
» 8 wheat crackers
» Sliced tomato with 1 cup cucumbers, sprinkled with dill
» ¾ cup blueberries
» 1 cup fat-free yogurt
» Herbal tea or other calorie-free beverage

Dinner
» Grilled chicken and vegetable kebabs: Marinate 3 ounces chicken in pineapple juice. Skewer and grill chicken pieces, bell peppers, cherry tomatoes and ½ cup pineapple chunks.
» ⅔ cup brown rice, tossed with parsley
» 2 cups spring greens with ½ cup orange segments and light vinaigrette
» Green tea or other calorie-free beverage

Snack (anytime)
» 2 ounces (½ cup) unsalted pretzel twists
» ½ cup plain yogurt with dill (dip)

Menu 2 nutritional analysis
Food servings
Grain/carbohydrate: 7
Fruits: 4
Vegetables: 6
Protein/dairy: 7
Fats: 3
Sweets: 1

Nutrient content per menu
Calories: 1,800
Fat (g): 40
Saturated fat (g): 12
Cholesterol (mg): 300
Sodium (mg): 1,535
Calcium (mg): 1,400

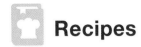

Recipes

Wild rice soup
Serves 6 (about 1½ cups per serving)

» 1 tablespoon margarine
» ½ cup diced onion
» 1 cup diced celery
» ⅔ cup sliced mushrooms
» ½ cup cubed turkey
» ¼ cup flour
» 4 cups low-sodium chicken broth
» ¼ cup fat-free dry milk
» ½ cup skim milk
» 1½ cups cooked wild rice
» Cracked black pepper to taste

Sauté onions, celery, mushrooms and turkey in margarine. Add flour and stir well. Add chicken broth, dry milk and skim milk, stirring constantly. Add cooked wild rice. Simmer. Season with cracked black pepper.

Nutritional analysis
Food servings

Grain/carbohydrate: ½
Vegetable: ½
Protein/dairy: ½
Fat: 1

Nutrient content per serving
Calories: 150
Fat (g): 4
Saturated fat (g): 1
Cholesterol (mg): 15
Sodium (mg): 165
Calcium (mg): 75

Chocolate ricotta mousse
Serves 6 (generous ½-cup portions)

» 3 ounces unsweetened chocolate, melted
» 1 pound part-skim ricotta cheese
» 1 teaspoon vanilla
» ⅓ cup honey

Blend melted chocolate, ricotta cheese, vanilla and honey in a blender or food processor until very smooth. Pour mixture into dessert cups and chill. To serve, garnish each serving with a fresh ripe strawberry, a few raspberries, or an orange or kiwi slice.

Nutritional analysis
Food servings

Protein/dairy: 1
Fats: 2

Nutrient content per serving
Calories: 235
Fat (g): 13
Saturated fat (g): 4
Cholesterol (mg): 23
Sodium (mg): 105
Calcium (mg): 220

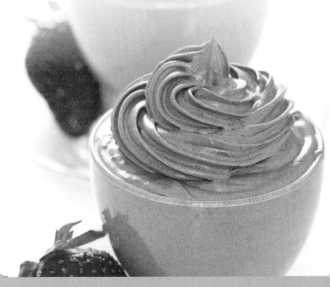

Tropical smoothie
Serves 4

- » 1 cup light, fat-free vanilla yogurt
- » 1 cup calcium-fortified orange juice
- » 1 banana
- » ½ cup crushed unsweetened pineapple

Place all ingredients into a blender. Blend until smooth and serve. To make a thicker, chillier smoothie, freeze the banana and pineapple before blending.

Nutritional analysis
Food servings
Fruits: 1½
Protein/dairy: ½

Nutrient content per serving
Calories: 120
Fat (g): trace
Saturated fat (g): trace
Cholesterol (mg): trace
Sodium (mg): 30
Calcium (mg): 195

Spinach with feta cheese and almonds
Serves 6 (generous ½-cup portions)

- » ¼ cup slivered almonds
- » 1 teaspoon extra-virgin olive oil
- » 1 large garlic clove, chopped
- » 4 scallions, or green garden onions with tops, chopped
- » 1½ pounds spinach, stems removed and well-washed in several changes of cold water
- » A small amount of water
- » Freshly ground black pepper
- » 4 ounces crumbled, reduced-fat feta cheese, at room temperature
- » Lemon wedges

Toast slivered almonds in a sauté pan over medium heat until slightly browned and fragrant. Put aside to cool. In the same pan, heat oil, add garlic and scallions, and cook gently for 15 to 20 seconds, being careful not to let the garlic brown. Add spinach and a bit of water. Cover and cook for about 1 minute. The spinach will wilt rapidly. Remove from heat and top with black pepper, feta cheese crumbles and toasted almonds. Garnish with lemon wedges and serve immediately.

Nutritional analysis
Food servings
Protein/dairy: ½
Fats: 1
Vegetable: 2

Nutrient content per serving
Calories: 140
Fat (g): 9
Saturated fat (g): 2
Cholesterol (mg): 15
Sodium (mg): 300
Calcium (mg): 190

Milk myths

Got milk? Some people will respond by saying, "No way." Like many foods, milk has its critics. Individuals leery of milk express concerns about the health and safety of milk and other dairy products. Here are some common misconceptions about milk:

It makes you fat. To limit fat and calories, some people needlessly rule out all dairy products. The association between milk and body fat is controversial; however, regular consumption of low-fat versions of milk, yogurt and cheese can be part of a weight-loss diet.

It causes allergies. Milk allergies are usually a reaction to certain components in milk, such as the protein casein. Milk allergies are uncommon. About 1 to 3 percent of children experience allergies to cow's milk, which they usually outgrow by age 3. In adults, milk allergies are even more rare. On the other hand, lactose intolerance is fairly common, but most people with this intolerance can consume small amounts of milk or dairy products without experiencing symptoms.

It's full of antibiotics and hormones. The use of antibiotics and hormones in animal foods is controversial. The Food and Drug Administration has approved them, as well as the use of bovine somatotropin (bST) to promote milk production in dairy cattle. This hormone occurs naturally in milk and is biologically inactive in humans. Even so, you can buy milk made from cows not given bST — the packages are labeled to reflect this.

It weakens bones. Scientific research has shown that milk and dairy products are good sources of nutrients that are vital for strong bones. For example, several randomized, controlled clinical trials — the gold standard of medical research — that used dairy products all showed significantly positive effects on bone health.

Many people avoid milk and dairy products because of such misconceptions. Unfortunately, in doing so, they're depriving themselves of foods they may enjoy and that provide important nutrients, especially calcium.

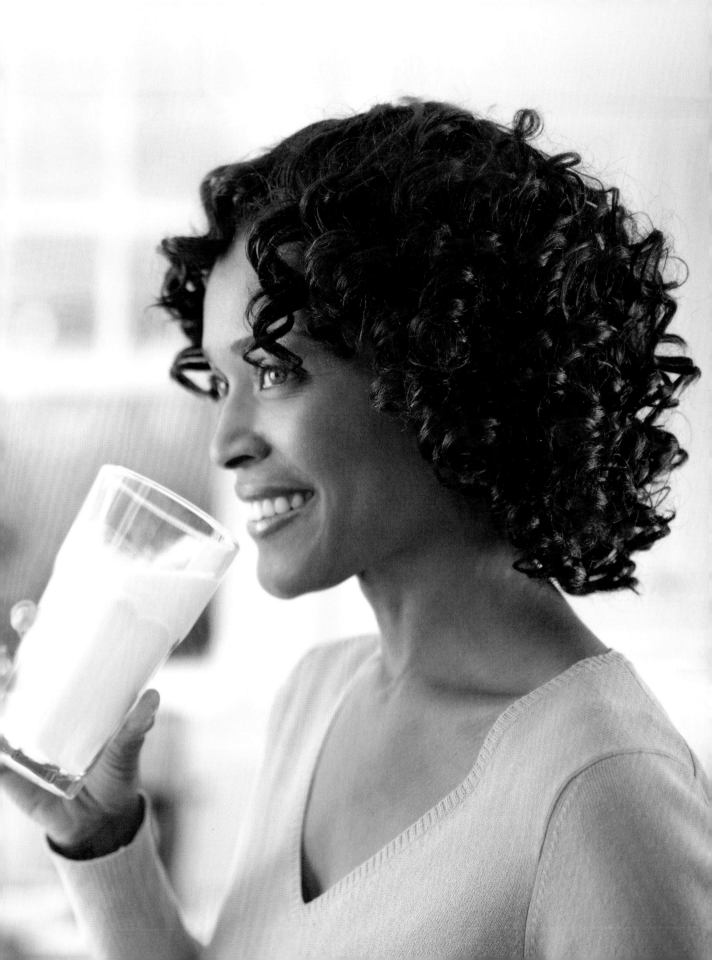

Increasing your calcium intake

Now that you know which foods are high in calcium, work on finding ways to make these foods part of your daily diet. Try to eat at least one serving of a calcium-rich food at each meal. Three servings a day can provide as much as 900 mg of calcium toward your daily goal of 1,000 to 1,200 mg. Consider the following tips:

- Add 1 ounce — a slice or two — of Swiss cheese to your sandwich for an extra 200 mg of calcium.
- Make soup with low-fat milk instead of water. A 2-cup portion of soup will provide about 300 mg of calcium.
- Prepare instant oatmeal with low-fat milk instead of water — ½ cup of low-fat milk added to a packet of oatmeal provides about 150 mg of calcium. Fortified instant oats provide another 100 mg.
- Instead of sour cream, which has little calcium and lots of fat, dip vegetables and fruit into fat-free yogurt. Most varieties of plain yogurt have at least 450 mg of calcium per 8-ounce cup.
- Like Southern-style foods? One cup of each of the following has about 100 to 250 mg of calcium: cooked greens (turnip, collard, kale, beet or spinach), okra, black-eyed peas and white beans.
- When making a smoothie, substitute ½ cup of low-fat milk or yogurt for water or use ½ cup of calcium-fortified orange juice instead of plain juice to boost the calcium content. You may also mix in a tablespoon of malt powder (60 mg

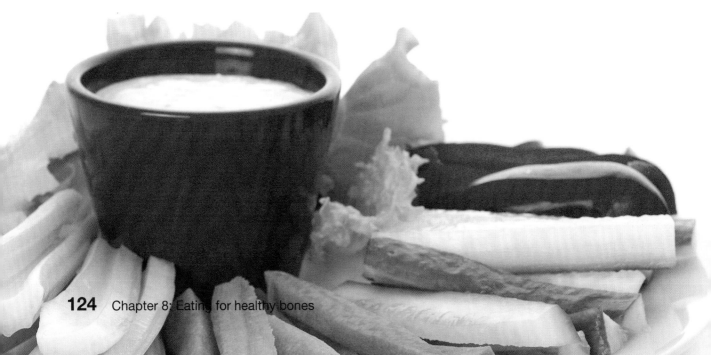

of calcium) or dark molasses (170 mg of calcium).

- Gourmet treatment can add a calcium punch to plain foods. Serve eggs or fish on a 1-cup bed of cooked spinach for about 250 mg of calcium. Or add 65 mg of calcium when you garnish vegetables or fish with 3 tablespoons of slivered almonds.
- Like Asian foods? Think soy. Many soy foods are a great source of calcium. These include *edamame*, the Japanese word for "fresh soybeans," which is commonly found in the supermarket with other frozen vegetables. One cup has about 260 mg of calcium. Firm tofu can be used in place of meat, poultry or fish in a stir-fry, with 860 mg of calcium per ½ cup. Snack on soy nuts, which are dried soybeans. One-third cup has about 50 mg of calcium.

When cooking, remember not to add milk to hot ingredients because milk scorches easily. Instead, add hot ingredients gradually to the milk, and then bring the whole mixture up to temperature. Most recipes containing milk can also be cooked without scorching in the microwave or in a double boiler. When using ingredients that are high in acid, prevent curdling by adding them to the milk gradually rather than vice versa.

Calcium supplements

If you aren't getting enough calcium in your diet, you may need a calcium supplement to make up for what you're lacking. A supplement is often recommended for postmenopausal women because calcium supplementation can reduce the rate of bone loss.

Types

Different kinds of calcium compounds are used in calcium supplements. Each compound contains varying amounts of the mineral calcium — referred to as elemental calcium. Common calcium supplements may be labeled as:

- Calcium carbonate (40 percent elemental calcium)
- Calcium citrate (21 percent elemental calcium)
- Calcium gluconate (9 percent elemental calcium)
- Calcium lactate (13 percent elemental calcium)

The two main forms of calcium supplements are carbonate and citrate. Calcium carbonate is cheapest and therefore often a good first choice. Other forms of calcium in supplements include gluco-nate and lactate.

In addition, some calcium supplements are combined with vitamins and other minerals. For instance, some calcium supplements may also contain vitamin D or magnesium. Check the ingredient list to see which form of calcium your calcium supplement is and what other nutrients it may contain. This information is important if you have any health or dietary concerns.

Choosing a supplement

To determine which calcium supplement may be best for you, consider these factors.

Amount of calcium

Elemental calcium is key because it's the actual amount of calcium in the supplement. It's what your body absorbs for bone growth and other health benefits. The Supplement Facts label on calcium supplements is helpful in de-

Lactose intolerance

Does milk or ice cream upset your stomach sometimes? You may have lactose intolerance — the inability to fully digest the sugar in milk (lactose) and other dairy products. Signs and symptoms of lactose intolerance may include bloating, cramping, gas, diarrhea and nausea. Discomfort usually begins 30 minutes to two hours after ingesting foods that contain lactose.

If you're lactose intolerant, you still need calcium. And you probably don't need to forgo dairy products completely. Many people with lactose intolerance can comfortably digest a glass of milk with a meal. And people who can't tolerate milk often have no problem with hard cheeses, yogurt and lactose-reduced milk. There also are tablets or drops that you can purchase that can be chewed or added to milk to improve your tolerance to lactose.

If you prefer not to consume dairy products, you can meet your daily calcium needs with calcium-fortified foods and calcium supplements.

termining how much calcium is in one serving. As an example, calcium carbonate is 40 percent elemental calcium, so 1,250 mg of calcium carbonate contains 500 mg of elemental calcium. Be sure to note the serving size (number of tablets) when determining how much calcium is in one serving.

Tolerability

Calcium supplements cause few, if any, side effects. But side effects can sometimes occur, including gas, constipation and bloating. In general, calcium carbonate is the most constipating. You may need to try a few different brands or types of calcium supplements to find one that you tolerate the best.

Interactions with prescriptions

Calcium supplements can interact with many different prescription medications, including blood pressure medications, synthetic thyroid hormones, bisphosphonates, antibiotics and calcium channel blockers. Ask your doctor or pharmacist about possible interactions and which type of calcium supplement would work for you.

Quality and cost

Manufacturers are responsible for ensuring that supplements are safe and claims are truthful. Some companies may have their products independently tested by the U.S. Pharmacopeial Convetion (USP) or Consumer Labs (CL). Supplements that bear the USP or CL abbreviation meet voluntary industry standards for quality, purity, potency, and tablet disintegration or dissolution. Different types of calcium supplements have different costs.

Supplement form

Calcium supplements are available in a variety of forms, including tablets, capsules, chews, liquids and powders. If you have trouble swallowing pills, you may want a chewable or liquid form.

Absorbability

Your body must be able to absorb the calcium for it to be effective. All varieties of calcium supplements are better absorbed when taken in small doses (500 mg or less) at mealtimes. Calcium citrate is absorbed equally well when taken with or without food and is a form recommended for individuals with low stomach acid (more common in individuals 50 and older, or if taking stomach acid blockers), inflammatory bowel disease or absorption disorders.

Supplement risks

Calcium supplements aren't for everyone. For instance, if you have a health

Examples of calcium supplements

Calcium supplement	Amount of elemental calcium per tablet (in milligrams)	Number of tablets to provide about 500 mg of elemental calcium
Calcium carbonate (40% elemental calcium)		
Calcid	200	2½
Extra Strength Rolaids	270	2
Miralac	420	1¼
Os-Cal 500+D	500	1
Caltrate+D	600	1
Calcium citrate (21% elemental calcium)		
Citracal Regular with Vitamin D	250	2
Citracal Plus Bone Density Builder	300	1⅔
Calcium phosphate, tribasic (39% elemental calcium)		
Posture-D	600	1

condition that causes excess calcium in your bloodstream (hypercalcemia), you should avoid calcium supplements. If you aren't sure if a calcium supplement is appropriate for you, talk to your doctor.

It's not definitive, but there may be a link between calcium supplements and heart disease. It's thought that the calcium in supplements could make its way into fatty plaques in your arteries — a condition called atherosclerosis — causing those plaques to harden and increasing your risk of heart attack.

More research is needed before doctors know the effect calcium supplements may have on heart attack risk.

There's similar controversy about calcium and prostate cancer. Some studies have shown that high calcium intake from dairy products and supplements may increase risk whereas another more recent study showed no increased risk of prostate cancer.

As with any health issue, talk to your doctor to determine what's right for you.

Too much calcium

Dietary calcium is generally safe, but more isn't necessarily better, and excessive calcium doesn't provide extra bone protection. In fact, if the calcium in your diet and from supplements exceeds the tolerable upper limit, you could increase your risk of health problems such as kidney stones, prostate cancer and constipation. Too much calcium can also lead to calcium buildup in your blood vessels and impaired absorption of iron and zinc.

If you take calcium supplements and eat calcium-fortified foods, you may be getting more calcium than you realize. Check food and supplement labels to determine about how much calcium you're getting each day. You want to achieve daily recommended amounts but not exceed the recommended upper limit.

Foods to avoid

In addition to learning what types of foods and food ingredients are good for your bones, researchers are also discovering food ingredients that can harm your bones. There are some foods and beverages you want to avoid or consume only sparingly.

Limit sugar, salt and phosphate additives

Foods containing sugars that are added during processing generally provide a lot of calories, additives and preservatives, but few vitamins, minerals and other nutrients. For these reasons, dietary guidelines often recommend that you limit processed foods and beverages.

In the United States, the No. 1 source of added sugar in the diet is soft drinks. Approximately one-half of the U.S. population consumes sugar drinks on any given day. Carbonated soft drinks are the most-consumed beverages, with an average of 44.7 gallons consumed per person, a year.

Most Americans also consume too much salt. The recommended daily amount is 2,300 mg, which is equivalent to about 1 teaspoon of salt. Most of this salt is found in processed foods. Studies show that high levels of sodium are associated with high blood pressure. In addition, too much salt increases the amount of calcium you excrete from your body when you urinate.

Phosphorus, in the form of phosphates, is used as an additive in many processed foods such as hot dogs, chicken nuggets, chips, processed cheeses and spreads, instant gravies, sauces, fillings and puddings, frozen products that are breaded, and cola beverages. Too much phosphorus in your diet can interfere with how much calcium is absorbed through your small intestine.

To limit your intake of sugar, salt and phosphate additives, check the labels on processed foods you buy at the grocery store. When preparing meals, use herbs, spices and fruits to flavor food.

Limit alcohol and caffeine

Alcohol supplies calories but few nutrients. It can be harmful for many reasons when consumed in excess, and some people shouldn't drink alcohol at all. If you drink alcohol, do so in moderation. Drinking alcohol with meals also slows its absorption.

Consuming more than one to two alcoholic drinks a day can hasten bone loss and reduce your body's ability to absorb calcium. Drinking alcohol with meals slows its absorption. Women planning to become pregnant or already pregnant shouldn't drink at all.

Caffeine can slightly increase loss of calcium during urination, but much of

the potentially harmful effect is due to caffeinated beverages too often being substituted for healthier drinks, such as milk. Moderate caffeine consumption — about 2 to 3 cups of coffee a day — won't harm you as long as your diet contains adequate calcium. You can help offset calcium loss to coffee drinking by adding a tablespoon or two of milk to each cup.

Chapter 9

Staying active

Like the rest of your body, your bones thrive on movement. That's why activity and exercise are good for bone health. During childhood, regular physical activity increases bone mass. It helps you maintain bone density as a young adult. And it can help offset bone loss as you age. Physical activity also helps improve your posture and balance, which in turn reduces your risk of falls. Beyond its bone benefits, physical activity keeps you healthy and strong, and it can give you more energy.

This chapter guides you on the path to a more active lifestyle. The exercises described on the following pages are designed to strengthen your bones while minimizing your risk of fractures. No matter what your age or condition, regular physical activity can be a simple, pleasurable part of your day.

Putting thoughts into action

You may have always known that exercise is good for you, but in the past you didn't have the time, the energy or the right equipment to exercise. Maybe you found exercise boring, or you were afraid of getting injured. The fact is, most adults don't get enough exercise. Only about 20 to 25 percent of adults meet recommended guidelines for aerobic and muscle-strengthening activities.

If you're at risk of osteoporosis or you already have it, it's even more important to find ways to fit physical activity into your life. You may be reluctant to exercise because of concerns about injury or pain. But avoiding physical activity only aggravates bone loss and puts your skeleton in greater jeopardy. Your goal is to make physical activity a routine part of your day.

Physical activity doesn't have to be a tedious chore requiring long hours at the gym, fancy workout clothes or specialized equipment. Routine tasks can be just as important as formal exercise.

Exercise is generally viewed as a structured, planned approach that's often measured or timed, such as doing 15 stretches or walking briskly for 30 minutes. Activity, meanwhile, refers to almost every motion of your body as you go about performing daily tasks and living your life. Spending a part of each day straightening up the house, shopping, mowing the lawn, walking the dog or gardening can contribute to bone strength when the activities are done on a regular basis.

Although the activities of daily living are vital to any action plan for osteoporosis, the needs and capabilities of one person are quite different from those of another. This type of activity will need to be assessed individually by you and your doctor.

The information that follows focuses on a simple exercise program to supplement the regular activities in your day. It's hoped that a few general rules and tips will allow almost anyone, regardless of his or her specific circumstance, to establish a safe exercise routine. Several of the exercises described in this chapter may appeal to you and be included in your routine, but many other exercises would be suitable choices, too.

Getting started

If you're trying to prevent or treat osteoporosis, the types of activities and exercises you choose to do will be based on your goals, overall health status, degree of bone loss and what you enjoy doing. You may want to avoid some exercises and movements that could cause more damage to your bones. What's appropriate for one individual may not help another. Your doctor can help you determine what exercises will do you the most good and how intensely to do them.

The important thing is to participate safely in some activity in a regular and sustained manner. Any safe exercise is better than no exercise. Your best bet is to choose exercises that you enjoy. That way you're likely to stay active for the long haul.

Often a combination of different exercises is recommended to help prevent or treat osteoporosis. These include weight-bearing, resistance, and back-strengthening exercises.

Consult your doctor

If you have osteoporosis, talk to your doctor before starting an exercise program. For one thing, a doctor can assess your overall health status and family medical history, such as whether you or anyone in your family has or had cardiovascular disease or high blood pressure. Be aware that some medications, especially tranquilizers and those that help you sleep, can affect the way your body reacts to exercise. Ask your doctor about how your medications may affect your exercise plan.

You may also want to consult a physical therapist or an exercise specialist about appropriate exercise routines, including how best to warm up and cool down before and after exercise. A physical therapist can also demonstrate proper body mechanics, safe methods for stretching and strengthening muscles, and proper use of the equipment you use. Some hospitals and fitness centers offer special exercise classes for people with osteoporosis.

Assess your fitness level

Although some conditions, including osteoporosis, may prevent you from doing certain activities, almost everyone can participate in some form of exercise. It's helpful to have a realistic appraisal of your fitness level as you plan your routine.

If you can easily do all of your normal daily activities at a reasonable pace without becoming breathless or dizzy, breaking into a sweat, or having chest pain, you're probably fit enough for a simple exercise program. But keep in mind that other components of fitness, such as flexibility and muscle strength, also are important.

Signs of not being fit (deconditioning) include feeling tired most of the time, being unable to keep up with the pace of others your age, avoiding activities because you know you'll tire quickly, and becoming short of breath or fatigued after walking a short distance.

If you've been inactive or in a weakened condition or you have low bone density, don't expect to be able to run 3 miles and lift heavy weights. And don't plan to work out two hours a day, 365 days a year. Begin with short amounts of physical exercise — per-

haps no more than five to 10 minutes. If all goes well, begin to gradually increase your activity. Try to keep physical exertion at a level you can safely and comfortably perform.

Set your goals

Setting goals is a good way to get motivated and stick with your exercise program. Try to make your goals realistic and achievable. It's always encouraging to see or feel some results as you exercise. Setting your goals too high can lead to frustration and failure.

Your physical activity goals may center around:

- Increasing your ability to carry out daily tasks and activities
- Maintaining or improving your posture and balance
- Relieving or lessening pain
- Preventing falls and fractures
- Increasing your sense of well-being

If you have chronic pain, your goals also may include exercises to help lessen your pain and increase mobility. After consulting with your doctor or physical therapist, you may come up with a list of several gentle stretches to try. Perhaps your initial goal will be to

Warning signs during exercise

No matter what exercise you're doing, stop and seek immediate care if you experience any of these warning signs:

- Tightness in your chest
- Severe shortness of breath
- Chest pain or pain in your arms or jaw, especially on the left side
- Heart palpitations
- Dizziness, faintness or feeling sick to your stomach

do a certain number of stretches each day for a week. At the end of the week, note whether your pain has lessened and whether you're able to move a bit more easily. If so, consider increasing your activity — adding a short walk to your day or increasing the number of stretching exercises you do. If you're not feeling better, talk to your doctor about other possible exercises.

If your overall goal is to improve your posture, perhaps start with a few balance and posture exercises every other day. Or maybe your goal is to walk briskly for 30 minutes, four days a week. Start with 10 to 15 minutes daily and build from there.

It's important to monitor your activity and adapt what you do so that it serves you best. You might want to keep an exercise diary to chart your progress.

Avoid risky movements

If you have low bone density or already have osteoporosis, a few precautions may be necessary when you exercise or perform physical activities. Certain movements may be dangerous because of the stress they put on the spine. This includes some positions used in yoga. Yoga positions that involve severe flexing or twisting of the spine may lead to compression fractures.

You may not be able to avoid all movements that can potentially be dangerous. Practicing good posture and body mechanics and paying attention to how you move will help.

Forward bending
Avoid activities and exercises that involve bending forward because they

increase the risk of compression fractures of your vertebrae. Try not to let your back bend forward as you make the bed, tie your shoes, pull weeds, reach down to pick up something from the floor and other such activities. Instead, keep your back straight as you bend at the knees to lower your body. Forward bending of the torso is especially dangerous if you're carrying anything, such as when you take a heavy pan out of the oven or set a bag of groceries on the floor.

Heavy lifting

Avoid heavy lifting, which may include loads of laundry, bags of groceries or exercise weights. This lifting will increase the stress on your vertebrae. If you must lift a heavy object, carry it close to your body. Be careful about opening windows or a garage door.

Twisting

Twisting movements can place unusual force on the spine. When you're driving, use your side mirrors for backing up and parking so that you avoid twisting to look through the rear window. Golfing and bowling are two common sports that involve twisting and may be harmful. Talk to your doctor or physical therapist about whether you can safely participate in these activities.

Reaching overhead

Reaching above your shoulders, as happens when you reach for something on the top shelf of the kitchen cupboard, isn't recommended for people with severe stooped posture.

High-impact activities

Activities that involve jarring movements, sudden stops and starts, and abrupt weight shifts put too much stress on the spine and can lead to falls and knee injuries in older adults. These include jogging, running, soccer, racket sports, volleyball and basketball.

Do it!

A big challenge that many people face when it comes to exercise is finding the motivation to stick with an exercise program. To be successful, you need to make a commitment to being active. This doesn't mean that you won't have setbacks or occasionally need to take breaks. The key is to keep going. Consider these tips:

- **Start slowly.** Don't jump into an intense exercise program right away if you haven't been physically active. Focus on small amounts of activity and gradually work up to more strenuous forms of exercise.

Low-impact weight-bearing activities

Any of the following activities would generally be a safe, invigorating choice for someone with osteoporosis:

- Walking
- Treadmill walking
- Using an elliptical machine
- Using a stair-step machine
- Low-impact aerobics
- Dancing
- Light gardening
- Deep-water walking
- Water aerobics

Water activities don't provide the impact your bones need to slow mineral loss, but they can be beneficial for individuals with severe osteoporosis.

- **Schedule exercise into your day.** Schedule exercise into your day just as you would an important errand or a social event. But don't be rigid about sticking to your schedule if you don't feel up to it. If you're very tired or you're under the weather, take a day or two off.
- **Pace yourself.** If you're unable to talk while you're exercising, you're probably working too hard. Slow your pace.
- **Listen to your body.** You may feel some muscle soreness and discomfort as you begin exercising, but you shouldn't feel pain and the soreness shouldn't last more than 24 to 48 hours. If the discomfort persists, you may be working too hard and need to ease up.

Exercises for osteoporosis

Three types of exercise are often recommended for people with osteoporosis: back-strengthening exercise, weight-bearing exercise and resistance exercise. Doing a little of each in a structured program can help you keep your bones strong and maintain good posture. Remember that exercise doesn't have to be strenuous or high impact to be effective.

Warming up and cooling down

It's important to allow time for warming up before any physical exercise and cooling down afterward. Warming up gradually increases your heart rate, and it limbers up your muscles, which reduces your risk of injury.

To warm up, walk slowly, then increase your pace gradually. Or begin an activity, such as bicycling or swimming, at a slower pace than what you're accustomed to until you feel loose.

End each exercise session by walking slowly or by continuing to do the activity at a slower pace. It's also a good time to stretch the muscles you used during your exercise.

Weight-bearing exercise

Weight-bearing exercises have nothing to do with weightlifting equipment. They're done on your feet with the bones of your lower body supporting your own weight. These activities help slow mineral loss in the bones of your legs, hips and lower spine.

Many young adults build bone mass through their participation in high-impact activities, which places greater loads on their bones. High-impact activities include jogging, soccer, basketball, volleyball, racket sports, gymnastics, dance and figure skating.

Older adults or people with low bone density should take precautions against too much impact and avoid activities that involve a high risk of falling. Low-impact activities such as walking place less stress on fragile bones.

Someone in a frail condition may opt for weight-supported exercises — as opposed to weight-bearing exercises. Weight-supported exercises include swimming, floor exercises or cycling on a stationary bike.

Walking: An ideal exercise

Walking is considered a safe, simple, cost-free exercise that causes minimal jarring to your bones. It requires no special equipment, lessons, other participants or membership fees. For many older adults and those with osteoporosis, walking is a mainstay activity.

A walking program shouldn't be too easy or too hard. When you start, walk a short distance at a comfortable speed. Then gradually increase your distance but not the pace. As you feel yourself becoming better conditioned, you can begin a more formal program of fitness walking. This requires a speed of around 3 to 5 miles per hour. A walking program should be done at least every other day to build both flexibility and endurance.

Remember that weight bearing is all about being on your feet. The most important thing is to choose exercises that you enjoy. Walking not only improves your balance and coordination, it's one of the best exercises for reducing your risk of falls.

Take a brisk walk around the block with a neighbor or walk on a treadmill while watching television. If you don't use walking as a form of regular exercise, fit in short walks whenever possible. Make your walks more fun by bringing a friend or your spouse. On poor-weather days, consider indoor walking at a mall or a health club. Remember to include warm-up and cool-down periods.

Aerobic benefits

Weight-bearing exercises also provide aerobic benefits. Aerobic activities increase your breathing and heart rates, which improve the health of your heart, lungs and circulatory system. This gives you more stamina and endurance, which make it easier to do whatever you need to do, whether it's cleaning the house or climbing the bleachers at your granddaughter's basketball game.

Even if your doctor advises you to avoid weight-bearing exercises, you can still gain aerobic benefits from low- or no-impact exercises, such as swimming, water exercises and indoor cycling.

Resistance exercises

Whereas weight-bearing exercise uses gravity to strengthen the bones in your lower body, resistance exercise applies weight — or resistance — to specific muscles to strengthen them. Strong muscles allow you to stand up straight and move more assuredly, and they help keep you from falling. Activities that build muscle strength also work directly on bone to slow mineral loss.

To create resistance, your muscles have to push or pull against an opposing force. A common way to do resistance exercise is to lift weights, either with free weights or with weight machines. For this reason, resistance exercise is sometimes called weightlifting, weight training or strength training. But conditions such as osteoporosis make it difficult, if not impossible, to hoist heavy weights. Other, more gentle methods of resistance training include isometric exercises, resistance bands and water workouts.

Why do you need resistance exercise? As you grow older, your muscle fibers shrink in number and size. Sometime after age 30, your muscle mass begins to diminish by about 1 percent each year. That means you could be 40 percent weaker at age 70 than you were at age 30. Losing muscle mass not only

saps your strength but also affects your balance and coordination.

If you have osteoporosis, you'll need assistance in designing a resistance-training program that includes proper lifting techniques and that's appropriate for your degree of bone loss. Consult your doctor, a rehabilitation specialist (physiatrist), a registered physical therapist or a certified athletic trainer to determine the type of resistance exercise that's best for you.

Weight training

With proper supervision, many older adults, including those with osteoporosis, can participate in weightlifting. But you'll need to check with your doctor first. He or she can prescribe exercises based on your bone density and fitness level. The weights should be light. And you'll need to pay strict attention to proper technique to avoid placing too much stress on the spine.

Exercising with free weights is a great way to build muscle mass because it can simulate motions you make in real life, like carrying boxes or lifting a bag of groceries. Start with weights of 1 or 2 pounds — and not more than 5 pounds. You should be able to lift the weights comfortably at least eight times. One set of 10 lifts can build muscle.

Free weights and weight machines can be found at most gyms and health clubs and in some schools. You can make your own weights by filling old socks with beans or pennies or by partially filling a half-gallon jug with water or sand. Used weights also can be purchased by the pound at some athletic equipment stores. Make sure you receive instruction on how to use them.

Isometric exercise

These exercises involve tensing your muscles while holding them in stationary positions. When you push your arm against a wall, for example, there's a buildup of tension in the muscles even though your arm isn't moving. Your own body creates the resistance.

Isometric exercises are especially useful for people recovering from injuries that limit range of motion. You should avoid isometric exercises if you have high blood pressure or heart disease because your blood pressure can rise significantly during the muscle contractions.

Resistance bands

Large elastic or latex bands — they look just like large rubber bands — provide resistance when you pull on them. These exercise bands are made with different degrees of resistance to match your fitness level. Consult your doctor or an exercise specialist to select an appropriate resistance level. Someone with osteoporosis should start exercising with low-resistance bands. Resistance bands can easily be used at home or packed in a suitcase when you travel. Some bands have handles or an anchor so that they can be attached to a door.

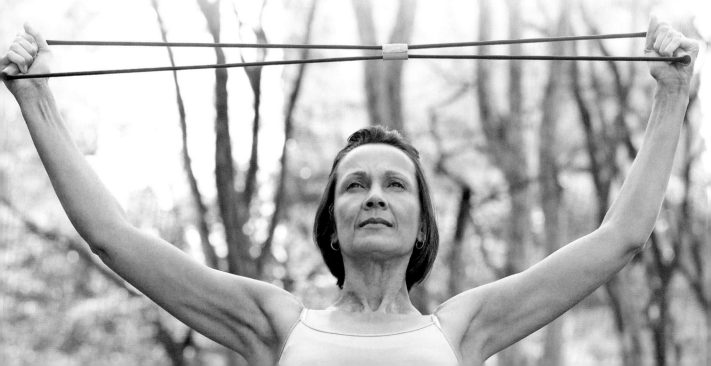

Water workouts

Water offers resistance as you push against it. Simply walking in water using correct posture will strengthen your abdominal muscles. You can also perform upper and lower body moves such as curls and squats in the water. For a more intense workout, use barbells and weighted boots, which add to water's natural resistance.

Many organizations, including YMCAs, YWCAs, health clubs and hospitals, offer water exercise classes. Be sure to inform your instructor if you have any health conditions such as osteoporosis that might affect your workout.

Whole-body vibration

With whole-body vibration, you stand, sit or lie on a machine with a vibrating platform. As the machine vibrates, it transmits energy to your body.

The low-intensity vibrations generated by the machine are said to mimic the effects of weight-bearing exercises. They make muscles work against gravity, thereby stressing bones enough to cause them to rebuild themselves and, theoretically, increase their density.

Whole-body vibration may offer some fitness and health benefits, but it's not clear if this type of activity is as good

Resistance exercises

Following are some simple resistance exercises that you can try. Move slowly and smoothly as you perform each of these exercises. Inhale before you lift or exert, and exhale as you lift.

To begin with, do three to 10 repetitions of each exercise. Take it easy and don't overdo it. Gradually add new exercises or more repetitions when, for at least three days, the original set of exercises becomes easy.

These exercises shouldn't hurt in any way while you're doing them or cause soreness for more than a day afterward. If they do, stop the exercises and consult your doctor or a physical therapist.

Resistance exercises are an important part of your exercise program because they can slow or even reverse age-related decline in muscle mass and bone density. They can also help improve compression fractures and stooped posture and reduce your risk of falls.

A doctor or physical therapist can provide instruction on additional exercises you can perform at home or the gym to help build bone mass.

Wall push-ups

Face the wall, standing far enough away so that you can place your palms on the wall with your elbows slightly bent. Keeping your heels flat on the floor, slowly bend your elbows and lean toward the wall, supporting your weight with your arms. Try to keep your back straight. Straighten your arms and return to an upright position.

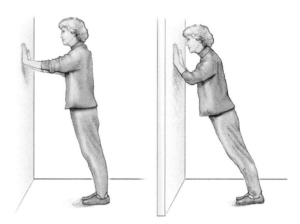

Chair sit-ups

Sit in a chair that has arms. Push your body up from the chair using only your arms. Hold this position for 10 seconds. Relax and repeat.

Biceps curls

Sit in a chair and have 1- or 2-pound weights in each hand. Start with your arms at your sides. Bend one arm at the elbow, lifting a weight to your shoulder without moving your shoulder or upper arm. Lower it slowly. Repeat with the other arm.

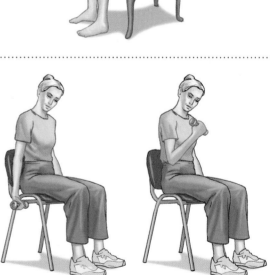

© MFMER

Back-strengthening exercises

Strengthening your back muscles can help treat osteoporosis by improving posture and reducing your risk of vertebral fractures. A few back-strengthening exercises are shown here. To begin with, try to do at least three repetitions of each exercise, but not more than 10. Add more repetitions when the exercises become easy. Remember to avoid exercises that round your back and increase pressure on your spine.

Talk to your doctor or a physical therapist about other exercises that help strengthen the back. Exercises that use specially designed, weighted backpacks may be beneficial in improving back strength and reducing compression fractures.

Lower back extensions

Starting from a hands-and-knees position, raise one leg at the hip, keeping your knee bent. Keep your trunk straight. Maintain this position for five seconds. Repeat the exercise with the other leg.

Upper back extensions

Sit upright in a chair. Put your hands on your hips or behind your back and squeeze your shoulder blades together. Hold the position for five seconds. Relax and repeat.

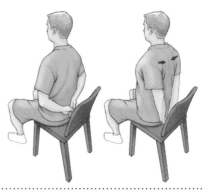

Pelvic tilts

Lie on the floor on your back with your knees bent and your feet resting flat on the floor. Tighten your abdominal muscles as you roll your pelvis down, flattening the small of your back against the floor surface. Avoid using your leg and buttock muscles.

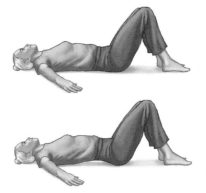

© MFMER

for you as regular exercise. Some research shows whole-body vibration can reduce bone loss as well as improve balance and decrease back pain, but comprehensive studies are lacking.

The device can also be dangerous. The vibration makes some people dizzy and faint, and some have fallen off the platform and been injured.

Because whole-body vibration can be harmful in some situations, check with your doctor before using it. You may find a whole-body vibration machine at a local gym or you can even buy one for home use.

How much exercise?

At this point, you may have a number of questions. How often should you exercise (frequency)? How hard a pace should you exercise at (intensity)? How long should you exercise (duration)? Your doctor or a physical therapist can help you answer all of these questions.

Remember that it's best to start out at a comfortable level and, when you're ready, gradually increase your exertion.

If you take more than a few days off, start back gradually — do less than you were doing when you last exercised. Here are some other tips.

Frequency

The more often you exercise, the better. To receive the maximum health benefits of exercise, try to do weight-bearing and back-strengthening exercises most days of the week. Include resistance exercise two to three times a week.

Intensity

For weight-bearing exercise, start at a pace you can continue for five to 10 minutes without feeling fatigued. As a rule of thumb, if you can't carry on a conversation while exercising, you're probably working too hard.

For most people, resistance exercise should be done at about 80 percent of their maximum muscle strength. This usually means lifting the same weight eight to 10 times. In general, to improve bone density and promote bone strength, the intensity of your activities — how hard you work — should increase over time. But the increase in intensity should be gradual.

Stretching and flexibility

Stretching exercises help increase your flexibility, another key component of overall fitness. Flexibility is the capacity to move a body part, such as a leg or an arm, in different directions around a joint, such as a knee or an elbow. Having a maximum range of motion around a joint helps prevent muscle injury.

The specific exercises you perform may depend on your physical condition and the exercise goals you've set for yourself. For example, for people with low bone density, the back-strengthening exercises described in this chapter may be useful.

Stretching exercises can be done every day, often in conjunction with weight-bearing exercise. The ideal time to stretch is when your muscles are loose — after you've exercised for eight to 10 minutes. Forcing muscles to stretch without a warm-up increases the risk of strains.

Stretches should be gentle and slow. Stretch only until you feel a slight tension in the muscle. Relax and breathe deeply while you stretch. Hold your stretches for at least 30 seconds. It takes time to safely lengthen muscles.

Duration

To begin with, try to accumulate at least 30 minutes of weight-bearing exercise each day. This doesn't have to be accomplished all at one time. Rather, it's the total amount of activity you undertake in a day, including routine tasks.

After a period of about six months — during which time you've gradually become more fit and increased your activity level — your daily routine might include a five-minute warm-up, 30 minutes of weight-bearing exercises and a five- to 10-minute cool-down period. Back-strengthening exercises may take 10 to 15 minutes. Two or three times a week include 10 to 20 minutes of resistance exercise. All of this activity can be broken into smaller sessions and spread throughout the day.

Staying in the game

For someone who's at risk of osteoporosis or already has it, activity and exercise play an important part in preventing or managing the condition. No matter what exercises you undertake, the important thing is to get moving and make physical activity a regular habit.

Your attitude is key. If you can't seem to stick with an exercise program, you're probably missing a crucial ingredient — fun. If exercise is drudgery, you won't do it for long. Make exercise part of everyday activities and hobbies that you enjoy. Be active with friends and family members or choose an activity you've always wanted to try.

Here are other ways to stay motivated:

- **If you're a beginner, develop a six-month exercise plan.** People who stick with a new behavior for six months generally have long-term success — exercise becomes a habit.
- **Choose exercises that fit your personality, physical health and lifestyle.** Do you like to exercise alone or with a group? Do you like being outside or indoors?
- **Add variety to your exercise routine to prevent boredom.** For example, alternate walking and bicycling with swimming or a low-impact aerobics class. On days when the weather is pleasant, do your back-strengthening exercises outside.
- **Join a class with people of a similar age and fitness level.** Peer support can keep you going.

- **Find an exercise buddy.** Exercising with a companion will help you stay motivated. Encourage your friends and family to be active with you.
- **Be flexible.** If you're traveling or especially busy a certain day, it's OK to skip or shorten your exercise program to accommodate your schedule.
- **Track your progress.** Keeping a log helps you work toward your goals and reminds you of how far you've progressed.
- **Reward yourself at milestones in your exercise plan.** Schedule something special that you've always wanted to do. Attend a concert or social event, meet with a friend, or go to your favorite restaurant.
- **Forgive lapses.** Everyone falls off the exercise wagon at some point. That's no excuse to quit. Remind yourself that it's just a temporary setback, and get moving again.

Keeping physically active on a regular basis is one of the most valuable gifts you can give yourself. Exercise can be as simple as a walk around the block or doing a few stretches while you listen to music. Being more active is one way you can take charge of your health and help manage a number of health conditions, including osteoporosis.

Chapter 10

Taking medications

Getting enough calcium and vitamin D in your diet and being physically active are key components of any plan for preventing and treating osteoporosis. But these measures alone can't completely offset bone loss due to aging and, in women, the onset of menopause. Diet and exercise also aren't sufficient to treat osteoporosis once you develop the condition. Medications are often prescribed to help slow bone loss and reduce your risk of fractures.

Your doctor may prescribe medication to prevent or treat osteoporosis in the following situations:

- You've been diagnosed with osteoporosis.
- You have low bone density, are postmenopausal or have other risk factors for osteoporosis.

- You experience continued bone loss or a fracture, even though you're physically active and get adequate dietary intake of calcium and vitamin D or are taking supplements.

The medication your doctor recommends will be based on a variety of factors. To date, there haven't been high-quality, head-to-head drug comparison trials to determine the efficacy of the individual drugs. Therefore, choice of medication is often based upon effectiveness, safety, cost, convenience and other factors.

For most postmenopausal women with osteoporosis, oral bisphosphonates are often the first line of treatment. Bisphosphonates are preferred because of their effectiveness and favorable cost and the availability of long-term safety data.

Hormone replacement therapy and osteoporosis

The hormone estrogen can help maintain bone density. However, the use of female hormones to treat osteoporosis — once a common practice — changed dramatically several years ago when the results of a study organized by the National Institutes of Health, called the Women's Health Initiative, were first released. The study was stopped early because it found a combination of the hormones estrogen and progesterone used long term increased the risk of breast cancer, heart attacks, strokes and blood clots in postmenopausal women. A few years later, another part of the study evaluating the effect of estrogen alone in postmenopausal women also was stopped early when it showed that long-term use of estrogen alone increased the risk of stroke.

Today, hormone replacement therapy is usually prescribed on a short-term basis to reduce the effects of severe hot flashes or other changes of menopause, such as mood swings or sleep disturbances, that are severe. The medication should be taken only for a short period of time and in the lowest dose possible. Hormone replacement therapy isn't recommended solely to prevent osteoporosis because other medications with fewer adverse effects have been shown to be equally effective. For women who cannot tolerate the other drugs, a short course of hormone therapy may be considered.

Hormone-related therapy

Newer medications that work in a similar manner to estrogen are sometimes prescribed to treat osteoporosis. Raloxifene (Evista) mimics the hormone's beneficial effects on bone density in postmenopausal women, without some of the risks associated with estrogen use. The drug may also reduce the risk of some types of breast cancer. However, hot flashes are a common side effect. Raloxifene may also increase your risk of blood clots.

Bisphosphonates

For both women and men, the most widely prescribed osteoporosis medications are bisphosphonates. Bisphosphonates inhibit bone breakdown, preserve bone mass, and even increase bone density in your spine and hip, thereby reducing the risk of fractures.

Bisphosphonates are anti-resorptive medications, meaning they work primarily by reducing the breakdown of bone tissue. The drugs alter the bone-surface actions of osteoclasts, the bone-excavating cells, and halt their functions. By doing so, bisphosphonates slow bone loss and increase the mineral content of bones.

Oral vs. infusion

Bisphosphonates may be taken orally in pill form, or they may be given intravenously. Oral bisphosphonates include the medications:

- Alendronate (Fosamax)
- Risedronate (Actonel, Atelvia)
- Ibandronate (Boniva)

These medications — which may be taken daily, weekly or monthly — generally increase bone density of the lumbar spine by approximately 5 to 10 percent. They also reduce the risk of new spinal fractures by 40 to 70 percent, and they reduce the risk of hip fractures by about 30 to 40 percent.

Oral bisphosphonates are often prescribed for postmenopausal women with osteoporosis, and they're generally the first choice of treatment for men with osteoporosis. Alendronate and risedronate are also approved for the prevention and treatment of glucocorticoid-induced osteoporosis.

The most common side effects of oral bisphosphonates are heartburn and abdominal pain caused by irritation to the esophagus or stomach. Taking the medications once a week or once a month doesn't appear to cause fewer stomach problems than does taking them daily.

Two bisphosphonates are available as infusion medications — drugs that are injected directly into a vein. One is zoledronic acid (Reclast, Zometa), which is administered once a year through an infusion. The other is ibandronate (Boniva), which is given as an infusion once every three months. The medications are typically administered in a hospital or at an outpatient infusion therapy center.

Taking bisphosphonates

Oral bisphosphonates may be taken in pill form once a day, once a week or once a month, depending on the medication. The less often the medication is taken, the larger the dose. Taking the proper medication once a week or once a month is just as effective as taking it daily and is more convenient for most people. However, a weekly or monthly dose doesn't appear to cause fewer side effects than does a daily dose.

For some people, oral bisphosphonates are hard on their digestive systems. If taken with a meal, with beverages other than water or with other medications or supplements, the drugs can bind to calcium- or phosphorus-containing compounds in the food, beverage or medication and leave the digestive tract without being absorbed. For this reason, bisphosphonates are taken on an empty stomach.

To help minimize any side effects, your doctor will recommend that you take your pill first thing in the morning with a full glass (6 to 8 ounces) of warm water. After taking the pill, remain upright — sitting, standing or walking — for 30 to 60 minutes to ensure adequate movement of the tablet through your esophagus and stomach and into your small intestine. Do this before eating, drinking anything other than plain water or ingesting other medications, including calcium supplements. Don't eat for at least 30 minutes.

Bisphosphonate medications administered by infusion don't cause stomach upset. The medications can be given anytime of the day.

Risks of long-term bisphosphonate use

Long-term bisphosphonate therapy has been linked to a rare problem in which the upper thighbone (femur) fractures. This injury, known as atypical femoral fracture, can cause pain in the lateral thigh or groin that begins subtly and may gradually worsen. It can sometimes develop in both legs at once. If such fractures show up on X-ray, therapy should be stopped.

Bisphosphonates also have the potential to affect the jawbone. Osteonecrosis of the jaw is a rare condition in which a section of jawbone dies and deteriorates. This occurs primarily in people who take very large doses of the medication by vein (intravenously) — much larger than the doses typically used for osteoporosis — because they have cancer in their bones. In these individuals, a small number have poor healing of the jawbone after a dental extraction or other trauma to the jaw. The risk of osteonecrosis of the jaw with regular use of bisphosphonates to treat osteoporosis is considered very small.

Because they don't cause gastrointestinal upset, intravenous medications offer an excellent alternative to postmenopausal women who may not be able to take oral bisphosphonates.

Which is better?

Both forms — pill or infusion — are effective. The type you receive generally depends on your personal preferences. There are some advantages to infused bisphosphonates. Researchers have found most women taking an oral bisphosphonate stop treatment or take less than the fully prescribed amount after one year of use. This reduces the effectiveness of the medication. An infusion given yearly or quarterly ensures that women are fully protected until their next treatment.

Some people who take several pills daily to manage other health problems don't like having to take yet another pill. And there are people who experience stomach upset from oral bisphosphonates. For these people, an infusion may be a welcome alternative.

Safety

Bisphosphonates have been studied for over two decades without any apparent serious side effects. The drugs generally aren't recommended if you have uncontrolled heartburn or gastro-esophageal reflux disease (GERD) or severely reduced kidney function. Your doctor will likely evaluate the safety and efficacy of the medications for your use on a yearly basis.

Bisphosphonates are also used to treat other bone diseases, such as Paget's disease, and bone affected by cancer that has spread from other organs. Bisphosphonates used for these disorders typically are given intravenously and more frequently.

In case of a fracture

Osteoporosis medications lower the chance of fracture, but they don't eliminate all risk of breaking a bone. If you have a fracture while on treatment, your doctor will reassess you to check for other problems that may have contributed to the broken bone.

Depending on the outcome of that assessment, you may be a candidate to switch to a more aggressive bone-building therapy such as parathyroid hormone, manufactured as teriparatide (Forteo). This treatment is typically reserved for women who are at very high risk — those with very low bone density or who have had fractures. Teriparatide has the potential to rebuild bone and actually reverse osteoporosis, at least somewhat.

Another option might be to switch to a newer type of osteoporosis drug called denosumab (Prolia). Denosumab produces similar or better results, compared with bisphosphonates, but works in a different way. It's delivered via a shot under the skin every six months.

Teriparatide

This medication is a chemical modification of the body's parathyroid hormone (PTH). Parathyroid hormone is produced by the parathyroid glands, which are located behind the thyroid gland at the base of your neck.

PTH plays a critical role in the bone remodeling cycle and in maintaining the calcium balance in your bloodstream. The hormone normally raises the calcium level in your blood in several ways. It releases stored

How long should you take bisphosphonates?

Bisphosphonates are considered safe and effective osteoporosis medications. But there's currently no consensus on how long postmenopausal women with osteoporosis or low bone density (osteopenia) need to take these drugs.

Up to five years of treatment with bisphosphonates is safe and effective. The scientific literature is full of good studies of all the bisphosphonate medications that prove their safety and show their effectiveness at preventing fractures of the hip and spine for up to three to five years.

Beyond five years of treatment, there's less certainty. One study shows that alendronate (Fosamax) — the most commonly prescribed oral bisphosphonate — improves bone density and reduces fracture risk for up to 10 years and is well-tolerated. Risedronate (Actonel, Atelvia) has been shown to be effective and well-tolerated for up to seven years of continuous use. Zoledronic acid (Reclast, Zometa) is considered safe and effective for up to six years of continuous use.

One thing that is known, though, is that even if you stop taking the medication, its positive effects can persist. That's because after taking a bisphosphonate for a period of time, you build up the medicine in your bone. Because of this lingering effect, some experts believe it's reasonable for women who are doing well on treatment — those who have not broken any bones and are maintaining bone density — to consider taking a holiday from their bisphosphonate after taking it for five years. But if you're at high risk of fractures or you have very low bone density, taking a break from your osteoporosis medication may not be a good idea.

So, what does this mean for you? Discuss your risk level and your options with your doctor to determine how long you should take bisphosphonates. Don't stop taking the medication without consulting your doctor.

calcium in your bones. It also increases calcium absorption by your intestines by stimulating production of a form of vitamin D in your kidneys, and it reduces the amount of calcium excreted by your kidneys. Although sustained increases in PTH can cause bone loss, intermittent increases of the hormone given by daily injection can strengthen bones.

The medication teriparatide (Forteo) is called an anabolic agent because it builds new bone. It works by stimulating osteoblast cells and, by so doing, increases new bone formation. All other medications currently approved for treating osteoporosis are anti-resorptive agents. They work by decreasing bone breakdown.

Researchers studying postmenopausal women with osteoporosis and a history of spinal fractures have found that daily injections of teriparatide, along with calcium and vitamin D supplementation, increased bone density of the spine and hipbone.

Teriparatide is approved to treat women and men with severe forms of osteoporosis, including those who are at high risk of fractures or who haven't responded well to other forms of treatment, such as anti-resorptive drugs.

Taking teriparatide

The medication is administered by a daily injection — which you perform yourself — in your thigh, hip or abdomen. Your supply comes in a disposable device that looks like a fat ballpoint pen. The device contains 28 doses — enough to last about one month — before it needs to be replaced.

Side effects

A warning that accompanies the drug states that one type of laboratory rat developed a small increased risk of cancerous (malignant) bone tumors called osteosarcomas after being given doses of teriparatide three to 60 times the amount given to humans. The large doses were given for the entire lifetime of the animals.

The Food and Drug Administration (FDA) reviewed this study and concluded that teriparatide is safe for human use because the chance of a similar problem occurring in humans is unlikely. To date, no humans treated with teriparatide have developed bone or other cancers due to the drug.

The optimal length of treatment with teriparatide hasn't been established. Because the long-term effectiveness and safety of the medication aren't known, the FDA advises that treatment should not continue for longer than two years. After two years a different drug is generally prescribed to help maintain the improvement in bone mass.

Teriparatide is quite expensive compared with other medications for treating osteoporosis. This limits the number of people for which the drug is a viable option.

Denosumab

Denosumab (Prolia) is used to treat osteoporosis in postmenopausal women who are at an increased risk of fractures, or women who cannot take or did not respond to other osteoporosis medications.

Denosumab is a monoclonal antibody — a laboratory-produced substance that inactivates the body's bone-breakdown mechanism. It's the first "biological therapy" to be approved for the treatment of osteoporosis. It works by blocking osteoclast bone resorption. In other words, it slows the bone-breakdown process. However, it also slows the entire bone remodeling process.

In one study, denosumab was given to women every six months for three years.

The women taking the medication were compared to women who received an inactive substance (placebo). Those on denosumab had a significantly reduced risk of breaking a bone, such as a spinal bone or hipbone, than did the women who received the placebo.

This medicine is also used in men to treat osteoporosis. The medicine may be prescribed for men who cannot take other medicines for osteoporosis or after other medicines haven't worked well. Denosumab injection is also used to treat bone loss in men and women who are receiving treatments for prostate and breast cancers.

Taking denosumab

The medication is delivered by injection every six months. This is typically done at a hospital or an outpatient infusion therapy center. The shot may be administered in the upper arm or abdomen but is usually given in the thigh.

Side effects

Common side effects of denosumab include skin irritation, back pain, and other bone, muscle or joint pain. Other side effects include high cholesterol levels and trouble with bone healing after a fracture or dental surgery. There have also been some cases of serious allergic reactions to the medication. People who have weak immune sys-

tems or take other medicines that affect the immune system may have an increased chance of having serious infections with denosumab. Even patients who have no immune system problems may be at higher risk of certain infections such as those of the skin.

Because denosumab lowers calcium levels, it's not recommended for people with very low blood calcium (hypocalcemia). Signs and symptoms of low calcium include spasms, twitches or cramps in the muscles; or numbness and tingling in the fingers, toes or around the mouth. However, most people with low blood calcium don't experience symptoms. Individuals receiving denosumab should also take calcium and vitamin D supplements.

Raloxifene

Raloxifene (Evista) belongs to a class of drugs called selective estrogen receptor modulators (SERMs). SERMs are sometimes referred to as designer estrogens because their chemical structure has been manipulated, or designed, in a laboratory. These synthetic compounds mimic some of estrogen's beneficial effects while avoiding some, but not all, of its adverse effects.

SERMs work by activating or inhibiting estrogen receptors in tissues that have these receptors, such as bone and breast tissue. Sometimes the drugs act just like estrogen, and other times they block the effects of estrogen. For example, raloxifene binds to estrogen receptors in bone cells, which may cause an increase in bone density in much the same way estrogen does. But when raloxifene interacts with estrogen receptors in breast tissue, the drug blocks the action of estrogen. This lessens breast cancer risk in women who don't have breast cancer but are at high risk.

Raloxifene was initially developed as a possible treatment for breast cancer and is similar to tamoxifen, another SERM used to prevent breast cancer recurrence. When researchers discovered raloxifene had a positive effect on bone density, their focus shifted to its use as a treatment for osteoporosis.

Raloxifene slows bone loss and prevents spinal fractures, but it's not as effective as other osteoporosis medications for preventing hip fractures. Among postmenopausal women with osteoporosis who didn't have previous fractures and who were studied for three years, daily treatment with the currently approved dose of raloxifene reduced the risk of vertebral fractures by 36 percent.

Among women taking a higher dose, risk was reduced by about 50 percent. However, treatment has not proved to significantly reduce other types of fractures, such as hip or wrist fractures.

Taking raloxifene

Raloxifene is available as a 60-milligram tablet. You take one tablet each day, preferably at the same time of day. It can be taken with or without food.

Side effects

Because of its anti-estrogen effects, the most common side effects with raloxifene are hot flashes. Conversely, because of its estrogenic effects, raloxifene increases the risk of blood clots, including deep vein thrombosis (DVT) and blood clots in the lung (pulmonary embolism.) Other possible problems include leg swelling due mainly to blood clots, bone pain and a flu-like syndrome. If these side effects are going to occur, they generally do so within the first few months of use.

Like estrogen, raloxifene increases the risk of blood clots by approximately threefold. However, the risk that an individual woman will have this problem is very low. If you have a history of blood clots or are at risk of developing them, your doctor may recommend that you avoid this medication.

Calcitonin

Calcitonin is a hormone produced in the thyroid gland. It doesn't appear to help regulate the amount of calcium circulating in the bloodstream, however, its function in humans isn't well-defined. During pregnancy and breast-feeding, the amount of calcitonin released by the thyroid increases considerably, protecting a woman's skeleton as her need for calcium increases.

A synthetic form of calcitonin is approved by the FDA to treat, but not prevent, postmenopausal osteoporosis. Like the bisphosphonates and raloxifene, calcitonin is an anti-resorptive drug, meaning it works by slowing bone breakdown. Calcitonin comes in two forms, a nasal spray (Miacalcin) and an injectable version. The nasal spray is the most commonly used form of the drug.

Calcitonin is safer but less effective than other medications for osteoporosis. For that reason, it's considered one of the last treatment options after bisphosphonates, teriparatide or raloxifene. Calcitonin may slow bone loss and modestly increase bone density. It's been found to reduce the risk of vertebral fractures, but it hasn't been found to decrease the risk of hip fracture. Calcitonin may also relieve bone pain in people with osteoporotic spinal fractures, especially in the first days to weeks after a fracture.

Calcitonin is generally used to treat women with osteoporosis who cannot take other medications. It may be prescribed for men who can't tolerate bisphosphonates, although it does not have FDA approval for this type of use.

Taking calcitonin

The nasal spray is administered by spraying one puff in alternating nostrils each day. The injectable form also is taken daily. The method is similar to injecting insulin for diabetes. The nasal spray and the injectable form of this medication should be refrigerated until opened.

Side effects

With the injectable form of calcitonin, side effects occur in about 20 percent of people who use it. They include nausea, irritation at the injection site, increased urination, and flushing of the face and hands. The only serious side effects of the nasal spray are nasal irritation and headache, which occur in a small percentage of people using the spray.

Thiazide diuretics

Thiazide diuretics are used primarily to lower blood pressure by reducing the volume of water in the body. But several studies have shown that thiazide diuretics can also increase bone density and prevent fractures. This may occur because diuretics reduce the amount of calcium that the kidneys excrete into urine. Because less calcium passes out of the body, more may be available for storage in your bones.

For people with high blood pressure, thiazides may be a good choice because they can help preserve bone density as they lower blood pressure.

Getting the most from treatment

In the last two decades, new medications for osteoporosis have helped to transform what was an insidious and unpredictable disorder into a treatable condition. The new medications hold promise not only in stopping the breakdown of bone but also in promoting bone growth, turning bone loss into bone gain. You and your doctor now have a variety of options from which to choose the most effective drug to fit your individual needs.

It's possible your doctor may also recommend a combination of medications. At least one small study indicated that a combination of medications — in this case teriparatide and denosumab — was more effective than either drug alone. Researchers still need to determine how long the drug combination remains effective.

No matter what drug you're prescribed, the key is that you take your medication as recommended. When you take an osteoporosis drug, you basically don't feel any different; you won't feel your bones getting stronger. For some people, this can make it difficult to stay on a treatment plan.

But it's important that you take your medicine if you want it to work. Taking an osteoporosis medicine half the time or less is the same as if you don't take it at all. Administer the drug — whether by pill, injection or a spray — just as your doctor prescribed. To get the most from your medication it's also important that you exercise regularly and get enough calcium and vitamin D.

If you decide that a particular treatment isn't right for you, express your

Drugs under investigation

Research is ongoing for several experimental treatments that may prevent bone breakdown or stimulate the formation of new bone. Investigators are looking for medications that are effective, easy to take, inexpensive and have few side effects.

Cathepsin K inhibitors
Cathepsin K is an enzyme produced by bone-resorbing cells (osteoclasts) that breaks down the collagen in bone as part of the bone-resorption process. Cathepsin K inhibitors reduce bone loss by reducing or blocking the action of this enzyme. Several cathepsin K inhibitors are being tested in clinical trials. One is soon expected to receive FDA approval.

Antibody to sclerostin
Sclerostin is a naturally occurring protein produced by certain bone cells. It plays a critical role in controlling bone mass by inhibiting the activity of bone-forming cells called osteoblasts. Antibodies to sclerostin are currently under study to see if they can block sclerostin and stimulate new bone formation by osteoblasts.

Vitamin D analogues
Vitamin D undergoes several conversions as it's processed in the body. Each conversion produces a new compound that's essential for the next conversion to take place. Various forms (analogues) of vitamin D used in other countries are being studied as possible treatments for osteoporosis in the United States. These compounds increase bone density in the spine, but their effect on fractures is unknown.

Growth hormone and growth factors
Growth hormone (somatotropin) is produced by the pituitary gland in your brain. The hormone plays a major role in stimulating bone growth during childhood and adolescence. It also affects bone remodeling in adults, but whether growth hormone can be used to prevent or treat bone loss is unclear.

Growth factors are proteins that promote skeletal growth, help repair body tissues and stimulate the production of blood cells. Laboratory studies indicate that they build bone, but they still haven't been fully tested in large clinical trials.

Others

Other new categories of drugs that stimulate bone development also are under investigation. Many of these medications are focused on certain signaling pathways that affect osteoblast formation.

concerns with your doctor. Don't just stop taking the medicine. It's important to see your doctor regularly and review your medicines at each visit. This will help to identify any side effects of the medicine and ensure that you're responding to treatment as you should.

To find out if and how well your treatment is working, your doctor may repeat your bone density test in a year or two. In some cases, doctors will also use special lab tests called bone marker tests, or biochemical marker tests, to monitor the effects of treatment.

It can take one to two years of treatment before significant changes in bone density can be measured with a bone density test. Bone marker tests, however, often can indicate if drug therapy is producing positive results in as little as three to six months.

Chapter 11

Osteoporosis in men

Osteoporosis is generally thought of as a woman's disease, but it can and does affect men. About 2 million men in the United States have osteoporosis and approximately 12 million more are believed to have low bone mass, putting them at increased risk of bone fracture.

At age 50, a man has about a 30 percent chance of having an osteoporosis-related fracture in his later years, and he has about a 6 percent chance of experiencing a hip fracture. Each year about 80,000 men break a hip.

Furthermore, men have a substantially higher disability and mortality rate after a hip fracture than do women. This is particularly true in the year immediately after the fracture. For men, the lifetime risk of an osteoporosis-related fracture is greater than the risk of prostate cancer.

The number of men affected by osteoporosis is expected to increase as more and more men live longer. In light of this, doctors and scientists are working to improve awareness of osteoporosis in men, and to provide accurate diagnosis and effective therapy.

Bone density in men vs. women

Women make up the vast majority of people who have osteoporosis — about 80 percent. Why is the disease so much less common in men? Several factors appear to account for the difference.

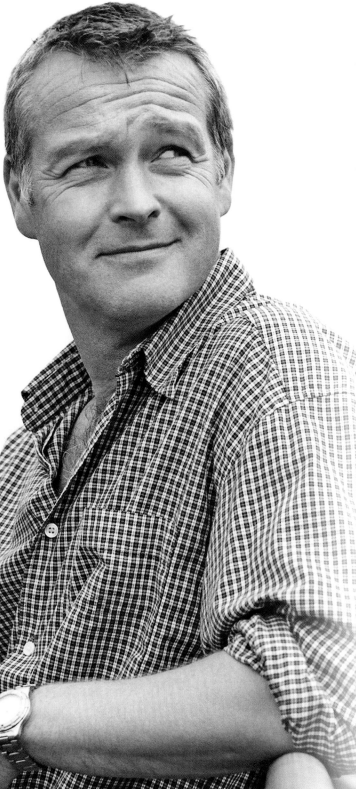

Higher peak bone mass

During puberty, bone mineral density in men increases substantially due to rapid increases in sex hormone production. Accumulation of bone mass peaks in a person's late 20s and early 30s for both men and women, but men typically achieve between 8 and 10 percent more bone mass than do women. This results in greater bone density due to bigger bones.

Bone density measured by volume is about the same in men and women in their 20s and 30s. But bones with a larger diameter give men an advantage when it comes to bone strength. There's more distribution area when forces are applied to bone, making it less fragile.

Lack of menopause

Like women, men experience loss of bone density as they age. But men don't normally experience a phase of rapid decline in hormone production, as women do during menopause. As a result, bone loss in men proceeds more slowly, unless a specific disease or disorder causes lowered hormone production, such as occurs with some types of prostate cancer therapy or certain hormone disorders.

Quality of bone loss

Bone loss in men and women that occurs as a result of normal aging mainly affects the spongy-looking inner core of your skeleton, called trabecular bone. In men, bone loss is characterized mainly by a thinning of trabecular bone tissue structure. In women, trabecular bone tissue structure becomes eroded and lost. In other words, trabecular bone structure in men remains stronger because it remains more intact than it does in women, even though the bone may be thinner than it once used to be.

How do men get osteoporosis?

Everyone loses some bone density with age, whether you're a man or a woman. After attaining peak bone mass, men start to lose bone density at a rate of about 1 percent a year. This rate of loss stays about the same throughout the rest of life. Beginning around age 65 or 70, men and women lose bone mass at roughly the same rate. This is because women have completed their rapid phase of bone loss by this age. During their lifetimes, men lose about 30 per-

cent of their bone density. If you're older than age 70 and are diagnosed with osteoporosis, it's likely that your age is a significant factor.

In about 50 percent of men with osteoporosis, the origin of the disease isn't due to an identifiable cause (idiopathic osteoporosis). Scientists suspect that men with idiopathic osteoporosis who are younger than age 70 have a genetic cause for their low bone density, and multiple genetic variations are likely involved.

In the other 50 percent of men, the disease is associated with one or more underlying conditions known to contribute to bone loss (secondary causes of osteoporosis). Most of these conditions also increase a woman's risk of bone loss. To find out more about secondary causes of osteoporosis, see Chapter 12.

Medications

Loss of bone mass is a common side effect of taking corticosteroid medications (glucocorticoids) used to treat conditions such as asthma or rheumatoid arthritis. Glucocorticoids appear to directly suppress new bone formation, but they may also disrupt vital hormonal processes. Other medications that may cause bone loss include anti-convulsants, chemotherapy drugs, hormone treatment for prostate cancer and excessive use of supplemental thyroid hormone medications.

Chronic illness

A variety of chronic illnesses can adversely affect your body's rate of bone remodeling, leading to bone loss.

Hormone disorders

Certain hormones play an important role in both bone resorption and formation. As a result, disruption of hormone production is a major risk factor for osteoporosis. This is why menopause affects a woman's risk of osteoporosis — her estrogen levels decline rapidly at this point.

In men, low levels of testosterone (hypogonadism), as well as estrogen, can increase the risk of osteoporosis. In fact, low levels of estrogen seem to be more strongly correlated with bone loss in men than are low levels of testosterone. Hypogonadism in men can result from several factors, including old age or certain hormone treatments for prostate cancer. Excessive production of parathyroid hormone (hyperparathyroidism) or thyroid hormone

(hyperthyroidism) also can increase a man's risk of osteoporosis.

Digestive disorders

Digestive disorders, such as inflammatory bowel disease, celiac disease and other malabsorption syndromes, can inhibit your body's absorption of calcium and vitamin D. These nutrients are essential to bone density and strength.

Other disorders

Other conditions that can increase your risk of osteoporosis include a disorder that causes too much calcium to be excreted from your body through your urine (hypercalciuria), chronic obstructive pulmonary disease (COPD), rheumatoid arthritis and certain cancers.

Lifestyle habits

Alcohol overuse or abuse may be associated with low bone mass or osteoporosis-related bone fractures, especially if the individual isn't eating well and isn't receiving adequate nutrition. Alcohol causes multiple effects on bone cells and is thought to mainly interfere with bone formation.

Smoking is another important risk factor. The specific cause and effect isn't clearly understood, but studies

Signs and symptoms of osteoporosis

In men — who, as a rule, aren't routinely screened for low bone density — the first indication of osteoporosis usually arises from one or more of the following signs and symptoms:

- A fracture that occurs with relatively little trauma
- Loss of height
- Hunched posture
- Sudden back pain

See your doctor if you notice any of these signs or symptoms. Unsuspected or untreated osteoporosis can make you vulnerable to a major fracture, such as in your hip, which can lead to loss of mobility and independence, and early death. The sooner low bone density is detected, the sooner treatment can start and the more effective such treatment may be.

show that men who smoke have less bone mineral density than do men who never smoked. Other personal habits known to increase a man's risk of osteoporosis include a sedentary lifestyle and low intake of calcium, vitamin D or both.

Genetics

Having a parent with osteoporosis — either your mother or father — is a major risk factor for osteoporosis in both men and women. By some estimates, more than half of all cases of osteoporosis are inherited.

Screening in men

Doctors continue to debate what groups of men would benefit from routine screening for low bone density — getting tested before any signs or symptoms are evident.

The International Society for Clinical Densitometry, which provides guidelines for the assessment of skeletal health, recommends that all men age 70 and older be tested for low bone density, even if a fracture hasn't yet occurred. In addition, most osteoporosis experts agree that men younger than age 70 should be screened in certain situations. These include:

- Signs or symptoms that suggest osteoporosis, such as back pain due to a low-trauma fracture, loss of height or a hunched posture
- Having an illness or taking medication that increases the risk of low bone mass
- X-ray results that incidentally show low bone mass or an unsuspected fracture

Getting evaluated

An evaluation for osteoporosis usually begins with a review of your medical history and a physical examination. In fact, if you have osteoporosis, your medical history and physical examination may provide an explanation for why the condition developed.

Bone density testing confirms the presence of low bone density. Your doctor also may order other tests — such as blood or urine tests — to determine whether an underlying condition may be causing your bones to weaken. Bone density testing is similar in both men and women. An instrument called a bone densitometer measures the mineral content of your bones in grams per square centimeter. The higher your mineral content, the more dense your bones.

A bone density test is usually done on those bones most likely to break, such as your lower spine, hip or wrist. One of the most common, and accurate, ways to determine bone density is with a dual energy X-ray absorptiometry (DXA) test. The test is usually done on your hips and lower spine. (For more information on bone density testing, see Chapter 5).

Interpreting the results

To interpret the results of a bone density test in a man older than 50, your doctor generally looks at your T-scores, numbers that indicate how much you deviate from the norm. The norm is the average bone density at a particular site — hip, spine or wrist — in a group of young healthy men at peak bone density.

For example, a T-score of 0.0 means your bone density is exactly average, compared with young healthy men at peak bone density. A T-score of -1.0 means you're one standard deviation lower than average, and a T-score of +1.0 means you're one standard deviation higher than average.

Similar to women, osteoporosis is diagnosed in men when your T-score is -2.5 or lower, and osteopenia when your T-score is between -1.0 and -2.5. (See Chapter 6 for more on testing.)

For a man younger than 50, your doctor generally looks at your Z-scores. These numbers indicate how much you deviate from the norm. The norm is the average bone density at a particular site — hip, spine or wrist — in a group of healthy men your age. For example, a Z-score of 0.0 means your bone density is exactly average for healthy men your age. A Z-score of -1.0 means you're one standard deviation lower than average, and a Z-score of +1.0 means you're one standard deviation higher than average. Similar to younger women, low bone density is diagnosed in a young man when the Z-score is less than -2.0.

Treatment

In many ways, treatment for osteoporosis in men is similar to that recommended for women. It generally consists of getting adequate calcium and vitamin D, regular exercise, and appropriate medications. If an underlying condition is contributing to your bone loss, your doctor will want to treat it.

Not all exercise is the same

For men with osteoporosis, experts recommend weight-bearing aerobic activities. These involve doing aerobic exercises on your feet, with your bones supporting your weight. Walking is a good example. Strength training exercises, especially those for your back, also can be helpful. Depending on the degree of your osteoporosis, your doctor may ask you to moderate or avoid high-impact sports, such as running or playing basketball, and exercises with twisting motions, such as golfing or bowling. For more information on exercising with osteoporosis, see Chapter 9.

Calcium and vitamin D

Getting enough calcium and vitamin D is a standard part of any treatment plan for osteoporosis, both for men and women. Calcium is one of the main components of bone. The amount of calcium you need to stay healthy changes over your lifetime. Your body's demand for calcium is greatest during childhood and adolescence, when your skeleton is growing rapidly. But older men also need to consume more calcium. As you age, your body becomes less efficient at absorbing calcium, and you're more likely to take medications that interfere with calcium absorption.

Experts recommend that men age 70 and younger get 1,000 milligrams (mg) of calcium daily. For men age 71 and older, the recommended amount is 1,200 mg. A daily intake of 1,200 mg also may be recommended for men age 70 and younger with low bone density or osteoporosis.

Getting enough vitamin D is just as important as getting enough calcium. Vitamin D improves bone health by helping calcium absorption. For individuals with osteoporosis or osteopenia, the Institute of Medicine recommends a daily intake of between 600 international units of vitamin D for adults up to age 70, and 800 international units a day for adults 71 and older.

Both calcium and vitamin D are found in vitamin D-fortified milk. Other dairy products, such as yogurt and cheese, are excellent sources of calcium. Foods rich in calcium include broccoli, spinach, salmon, and calcium-fortified juices or cereals. Sunlight is a major source of vitamin D; typically, all you need is 10 to 15 minutes of sun exposure — without sunscreen — twice a week to maintain optimum levels of vitamin D. In winter months when sun exposure is limited, supplemental vitamin D may be needed.

If you don't get the recommended amounts of calcium and vitamin D in your diet or from sun exposure, ask your doctor if calcium and vitamin D supplements are appropriate for you.

Regular exercise

Regular exercise can help maintain, and perhaps even increase, the density of your bones, making them stronger and less prone to fracture. Exercise also strengthens your muscles. Together, strong bones and muscles will improve your posture and balance, which can reduce your risk of falls.

A Swedish study involving more than 2,000 men — who at the beginning of the study were between the ages of 49 and 51 — set out to examine the influence that leisure physical activity might have on the men's risk of osteoporotic fracture. Over a follow-up period of 35 years, the researchers found that the more active the men were, the less risk they had of fracturing a bone. Specifically, hip fracture occurred in:

- 20 percent of men who lived sedentary lifestyles
- 13 percent of those whose activities included some walking and cycling
- 8 percent of men who participated in sports at least three hours a week

Even if you haven't been physically active, it's not too late to start. The researchers also found that men who increased their activity levels tended to lower their risk of fractures, whereas men who decreased their activity levels increased their risks.

Bisphosphonate therapy

Bisphosphonates — a group of drugs commonly used to treat osteoporosis — are effective in men as well as in women. Bisphosphonates work to inhibit bone breakdown, preserve bone mass and reduce the risk of fracture. They're a type of treatment known as anti-resorptive therapy. Once you start taking a bisphosphonate, the rate at which you lose bone mass slows more than the rate at which new bone is formed. Consequently, your bone density most often increases over time.

The Food and Drug Administration has approved three bisphosphonate drugs for treating osteoporosis in men: alendronate (Fosamax), risedronate (Actonel) and zoledronic acid (Reclast). These drugs are also effective for treating osteoporosis resulting from other conditions, such as long-term glucocorticoid use or hypogonadism. Alendronate is taken as a daily or weekly tablet. Risedronate comes in the form of a daily, weekly or monthly tablet. Zoledronic acid is given by infusion once a year.

Typically, you take bisphosphonates for up to five years. If you respond well to the therapy — meaning your bone density remains stable or improves and you experience no fractures — after five years your doctor may consider discontinuing the drug. There's evidence that the fracture reduction benefits of bisphosphonates persist for several years after therapy is ended. For more information on osteoporosis medications, see Chapter 10.

Teriparatide

Teriparatide (Forteo) is a shortened form of human parathyroid hormone that belongs to a group of drugs called anabolic therapies. Whereas anti-resorptive medications mainly prevent bone loss, anabolic therapies promote bone formation. Anabolic therapies also increase bone mineral density substantially in the spine, and to a lesser degree in the hip bones.

Teriparatide is approved for men and women at high risk of fractures, including individuals with a previous osteoporotic fracture, high risk of fracture due to very low bone density, or who haven't responded to other treatment. The drug is taken as a daily injection.

Because its long-term effects are still being studied, the FDA recommends restricting therapy to two years or less. After ending teriparatide therapy, your doctor may recommend bisphosphonate or other anti-resorptive therapy to maintain or enhance the bone density gained with teriparatide.

Testosterone replacement

If you have osteoporosis due to low levels of testosterone, such as occurs with hypogonadism, your doctor may recommend testosterone replacement therapy, alone or in combination with a bisphosphonate or other osteoporosis medication.

Testosterone replacement is shown to increase bone mineral density in men with low testosterone, but not in men with normal levels of testosterone. Evidence from clinical trials indicates that injected testosterone improves bone density in men with hypogonadism. Patches or gels containing testosterone haven't been evaluated thoroughly for this purpose, although there's no reason to think they should be less effective unless testosterone absorption is less than expected. Testosterone therapy isn't recommended if you have prostate cancer or are at high risk.

Self-care

In addition to proper medication, calcium and vitamin D supplementation, and exercise, you can also help reduce your risk of weak bones and fracture — and improve your overall health — with two other important steps. Quit smoking if you smoke, and limit your consumption of alcohol to a moderate amount. These lifestyle behaviors are also important to bone health.

Take action

Men generally believe that they don't need to worry about osteoporosis. Even though osteoporosis isn't as common in men as it is in women, it can be more disabling and more deadly if a major fracture occurs.

If you experience signs or symptoms of osteoporosis — a fracture from a low-trauma incident, loss of height or sudden back pain — don't ignore them. Talk to your doctor.

Even if you don't have any signs or symptoms, if you're older than age 70, you should have a bone density test as a preventive measure. In the long run, treating osteoporosis is a much better option than letting it go and suffering its potential consequences — a serious and disabling fracture.

Chapter 12

Disorders associated with osteoporosis

Most people are aware that osteoporosis is more prevalent with advancing age and, in women, the onset of menopause. Age and menopause are two common risk factors for the disease. However, they aren't the only two. Osteoporosis may develop for many other reasons. An underlying disease, a nutritional deficiency or a particular medication can increase your risk. Often, osteoporosis results from a combination of factors.

Having osteoporosis also may place you at increased risk of developing a related disorder, such as kyphosis, also known as hunchback.

This chapter looks at associated disorders — those that may increase your risk of developing osteoporosis or result from having osteoporosis.

Endocrine disorders

The body's endocrine glands include the pituitary, thyroid, parathyroid and adrenal glands. The pancreas, ovaries and testes also act as endocrine glands. The endocrine system controls cell activities by releasing chemical messengers in the form of hormones into the bloodstream.

A healthy balance of hormones is necessary to reach peak bone density and maintain bone health. In women, too little of the hormone estrogen can affect bone density in two ways. It can limit gains in bone density during growth and development, or it can increase the rate of bone breakdown and bone loss after the skeleton is mature.

In men, any condition that reduces production of the hormone testosterone can put a man at increased risk of osteoporosis. Low testosterone can limit gain of bone density during growth and development, or it can result in bone loss after the skeleton is mature. Too much or too little of other hormones also can affect bone health.

Following are some endocrine and hormonal disorders that can increase an individual's risk of osteoporosis.

- Hypogonadism, caused by decreased production of estrogen by the ovaries or testosterone by the testes
- Amenorrhea, a form of hypogonadism in which menstrual cycles are absent during a time in life when they should be present
- Cushing's syndrome, a condition in which the body abnormally produces too much of the hormone cortisol
- Hyperthyroidism, caused by excessive production of thyroid hormone
- Hyperparathyroidism, caused by excessive production of parathyroid hormone
- Type 1 diabetes, the form of diabetes in which the body no longer is able to produce the hormone insulin

Gastrointestinal disorders

Studies have found an increased risk of bone loss and bone fractures in people with certain gastrointestinal diseases or conditions.

Inflammatory disorders

Natural chemicals in the body produced by inflammation, such as occurs with inflammatory bowel disease (Crohn's disease and ulcerative colitis), are known to increase bone breakdown. In addition, certain medications used to treat some inflammatory gastrointestinal disorders, such as steroid medications, also increase bone loss.

Malabsorption disorders

People with malabsorption disorders, such as celiac disease, who are unable to properly absorb nutrients such as vitamin D and calcium may experience bone loss.

Bone loss may also occur as a result of weight-loss (bariatric) surgery in which part of the stomach and intestine is "bypassed" during digestion. The surgery can help an individual lose weight, but it can also reduce his or her ability to properly absorb bone-building nutrients in food.

Rheumatologic disorders

Rheumatic disorders include diseases such as rheumatoid arthritis, systemic lupus erythematosus and ankylosing spondylitis. Rheumatologic disorders usually result from autoimmune inflammatory diseases. An autoimmune disorder is a condition in which the body releases antibodies that attack healthy tissues.

With rheumatoid arthritis, for example, inflammation in a joint may result in the release of enzymes that can destroy the lining of the joint. Joints most affected are those in the hands, wrists, knees, feet and ankles. In addition to joint damage, people with rheumatoid arthritis and other rheumatologic disorders usually have lower bone mass than do individuals who don't have the conditions.

The reason why isn't clear, but it may be that certain inflammatory chemicals or chemicals produced by the diseased joints may also affect bone and lead to bone breakdown. In addition, certain medications used to treat rheumatic conditions, such as steroid medications, are known to increase the risk of osteoporosis.

Glucocorticoid-related disease

Glucocorticoid-induced osteoporosis is a form of osteoporosis that results from taking steroid (glucocorticoid) medications such as prednisone, prednisolone, dexamethasone or cortisone. These medications may be taken to help control asthma, emphysema, inflammatory bowel disease or a rheumatic disease, such as rheumatoid arthritis or systemic lupus erythematosus.

Glucocorticoid medications affect bone tissue in a multitude of ways. The medications have a direct negative effect on bone cells, slowing the rate of bone formation for as long as the medication is taken. They also temporarily speed up bone breakdown for several months after the medication is started. And they decrease the levels of the hormones estrogen and testosterone, which normally protect against bone loss. In addition, glucocorticoid medications affect how the body handles the mineral calcium — decreasing calcium absorption in the intestines and increasing calcium loss in urine.

Anyone who takes a significant dose of an oral glucocorticoid medication, or receives lower doses of an intravenous glucocorticoid medication, for more than three to six months is at risk of developing osteoporosis. Bone loss tends to occur most rapidly in the first six months after starting an oral steroid. After about a year of use, the rate of bone loss slows.

Steroids taken by mouth in the form of an inhaler may cause only mild bone loss and are preferred over steroid pills. Steroids taken in the form of a nasal spray don't appear to cause bone loss.

Bisphosphonate medications or the drug teriparatide is generally the treatment of choice for glucocorticoid-induced osteoporosis, along with calcium and vitamin D supplements. However, a recent study showed that teriparatide may prevent fractures more effectively than does the bisphosphonate alendronate in individuals taking oral glucocorticoid medication.

Other medications

In addition to glucocorticoids, a number of other medications may increase your risk of osteoporosis either by reducing peak bone mass (when the medication is taken during childhood or young adulthood) or by increasing bone loss later in life.

If you're required to take a medication associated with bone loss (see the chart on pages 182-183), talk to your doctor about steps you can take to help protect your bones.

Liver disorders

Osteoporosis is common among individuals with serious, chronic liver disorders. Liver disorders are thought to increase the risk of osteoporosis partly by decreasing vitamin D production, leading to calcium malabsorption. But it's likely that a number of other factors also are involved.

For individuals awaiting a liver transplant, glucocorticoid medications they sometimes need to take prior to their transplant surgery can lead to osteoporosis. It's also likely that chemical changes associated with liver disorders affect bone resorption.

In addition, chronic liver disease can reduce the production of male or female hormones, a condition called hypogonadism. Low estrogen and testosterone levels are known risk factors for osteoporosis. Excessive alcohol consumption associated with some forms of liver disease also is a risk factor.

Kidney disorders

Osteoporosis is common among individuals with late-stage chronic kidney disease. As kidneys begin to fail, the body begins to make increasing amounts of parathyroid hormone, which causes increased bone loss. The worse kidney function becomes, the worse hyperparathyroidism gets.

Failing kidneys are unable to make enough of the biologically active form of vitamin D, which limits the ability of the intestine to absorb calcium, aggravating the existing hyperparathyroidism. Chronic kidney disease often causes decreased production of male and female hormones, leading to hypogonadism. Because the kidneys normally clear toxins from the bloodstream, toxins may build up and cause bone loss by various means.

Transplant surgery

Many people who undergo an organ transplant take medications before and after surgery to help the body prepare for and accept the transplanted organ. These medications, which include steroid medications, certain diuretics, some blood-thinning medications and immunosuppressive drugs, can increase bone loss.

Often times, people undergoing an organ transplant experience end-stage organ failure before the transplant, which may cause bone loss. In addition, decreased physical activity due to fatigue associated with end-stage organ failure before a transplant may contribute to bone loss.

Cancer

Men and women with certain types of cancer are at increased risk of osteoporosis due to the effects of some cancers on the skeleton or to the medications and therapies required to treat the cancer. Treatments such as chemotherapy or therapy to reduce hormone production may decrease bone density.

Aromatase inhibitors are an important component of treatment for postmenopausal women with estrogen receptor positive breast cancer. The medications inhibit an enzyme responsible for the conversion of androgens to the hormone estrogen. Therefore, they cause bone loss due to estrogen deficiency.

Drugs and disorders associated with low bone density

Endocrine disorders
- Primary hyperparathyroidism
- Hyperthyroidism
- Type 1 diabetes
- Hyperprolactinemia
- Early menopause
- Cushing's syndrome
- Addison's disease
- Growth hormone deficiency
- Klinefelter's syndrome
- Turner's syndrome
- Acromegaly

Rheumatologic disorders
- Rheumatoid arthritis
- Systemic lupus erythematosus
- Ankylosing spondylitis

Gastrointestinal disorders
- Celiac disease
- Crohn's disease
- Pernicious anemia
- Malabsorption of any cause

Liver disorders
- Primary biliary cirrhosis
- Primary sclerosing cholangitis

Kidney disorders
- Chronic kidney disease of any cause

Medications
- Glucocorticoids
- Anticonvulsants (phenytoin, carbamazepine, phenobarbital or valproate)
- Levothyroxine (more than needed)
- SSRI antidepressants
- Cyclosporin
- Injections of Depo-Provera or steroids
- Diuretics causing hypercalciuria
- Long-term heparin therapy
- Lithium
- Methotrexate or other antimetabolites
- Antipsychotic medications (phenothiazine derivatives)
- Aluminum-containing phosphate binders
- Tetracycline (extended use)
- Gonadotropin-releasing hormone (Gn-RH) agonists
- Proton pump inhibitors

Genetic diseases
- Osteogenesis imperfecta
- Ehlers-Danlos syndrome
- Gaucher's disease and other glycogen storage diseases
- Homocystinuria
- Hypophosphatasia
- Marfan syndrome

- Menkes syndrome
- Mitochondrial myopathies
  Riley-Day syndrome
  (familial dysautonomia)
- Sickle cell anemia
- Thalassemia
- Congenital porphyria

Cancer
- Multiple myeloma
- Systemic mastocytosis
- Leukemia

Immobility
- Prolonged bed rest from any
  cause
- Spinal cord syndromes
- Prolonged space flight

Miscellaneous causes
- Vitamin D deficiency of any
  cause
- Low calcium intake or
  absorption
- Lack of physical exercise
- Pregnancy or lactation
- Alcohol overuse
- Idiopathic scoliosis
- Lactose intolerance
- Anorexia nervosa
- Chronic obstructive pulmonary
  disease
- Endometriosis
- Hemochromatosis
- Amyloidosis
- Epidermolysis bullosa
- Hemophilia
- Movement disorders
  (Parkinson's disease)
- Multiple sclerosis
- Prolonged parenteral nutrition
- Sarcoidosis
- Vegetarian diet

Because the medications can result in rapid bone loss, women receiving aromatase inhibitors to treat breast cancer should adopt lifestyle changes that promote bone health, including regular physical activity and a calcium-rich diet. In some cases, medication may be prescribed to help offset the loss in bone density associated with use of aromatase inhibitors.

Osteoporosis also is a side effect of certain therapies used to treat prostate cancer. Some men develop osteoporosis as a result of therapy to reduce hormone production, known as androgen deprivation. Bone mineral density screenings may be a good idea for men receiving hormone therapy. Steps that may decrease the risk of osteoporosis include exercise and adequate daily calcium and vitamin D. Medication to offset the bone-thinning effects of hormone therapy also may be prescribed.

Genetic diseases

A number of rare genetic diseases have been found to be associated with the development of osteoporosis. If you have one of the diseases listed on the chart on pages 182-183, be aware that your risk of osteoporosis is increased.

Kyphosis

Kyphosis is a forward rounding of the upper back. A certain amount of rounding is normal, but with kyphosis the rounding is more severe. While kyphosis can occur at any age, it's most common in older women. Other names for the condition include round back and hunchback. The deformity is also referred to as dowager's hump.

Age-related kyphosis often occurs after osteoporosis weakens spinal bones to the point that they crack and compress. A few types of kyphosis target infants or teens.

Mild cases of kyphosis may produce no noticeable signs or symptoms. However, severe cases can affect your lungs, nerves, and other tissues and organs, causing pain and other problems. In addition to an abnormally curved spine, kyphosis can cause back pain and stiffness in some people.

Certain groups of people are at higher risk of kyphosis.

- Adolescent girls with poor posture are at greater risk of postural kyphosis.
- Boys between the ages of 10 and 15 are at greater risk of Scheuermann's kyphosis.

- Older adults with osteoporosis are at greater risk of spinal fractures that can contribute to kyphosis.
- People who have connective tissue disorders, such as Marfan syndrome, also are at greater risk.

Treatment of the condition depends on the cause and the signs and symptoms that are present. Your doctor may suggest use of pain relievers. If over-the-counter medicines, such as acetaminophen (Tylenol, others), ibuprofen (Advil, Motrin IB, others) or naproxen sodium (Aleve) aren't enough, stronger pain medications are available by prescription. In addition, bone-strengthening drugs used to treat osteoporosis may help prevent additional spinal fractures that can cause kyphosis to worsen.

Other treatments for kyphosis include stretching exercises to improve spinal flexibility and exercises that strengthen the abdominal muscles to improve posture. Children who have Scheuermann's kyphosis may be able to stop the progression of the disease by wearing a body brace while their bones are still growing.

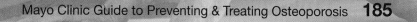

If the kyphosis curve is very severe, particularly if the curve is pinching the spinal cord or nerve roots, your doctor might suggest surgery to reduce the degree of curvature. The most common procedure, called spinal fusion, connects two or more of the affected vertebrae permanently. Surgeons insert bits of bone between the vertebrae and then fasten the vertebrae together with metal wires, plates and screws.

ity is observed in astronauts in space. When there's no gravitational stress affecting the bones, astronauts lose bone mass even though they may exercise to try to prevent bone loss.

Immobility

Any disease or disability that limits your ability to be active is likely to cause bone loss. Individuals who use a wheelchair or who have difficulty getting around are likely to experience a loss in bone density. They can't take part in weight-bearing activities or they have a hard time doing so.

Weight-bearing activities include any physical activity in which your feet or legs are supporting or carrying your weight. When you're immobile for a long period of time and you aren't able to walk or stand on your feet, you're at increased risk of bone loss.

An extreme example of what happens to bones without weight-bearing activ-

Part 3

Living with osteoporosis

Chapter 13

Healthy living strategies

Osteoporosis is a bone disease, but its impact extends well beyond your skeleton. Many people with osteoporosis learn how to live with the condition as they go about their daily activities. But for others, especially those who have fractured a bone, osteoporosis can take a tremendous physical, emotional and social toll.

If you have osteoporosis, work and household tasks may become more difficult and require assistance from others. You may experience pain and fatigue, as well as stress, anxiety and depression. Your social relationships may be more difficult to maintain, and you may not be as independent and active as you once were.

Coping with any chronic illness requires patience and perseverance. You don't have to give in to despair or avoid your normal routines. You can still maintain your quality of life.

This chapter presents strategies to help you cope with some of the physical, emotional and social aspects of having osteoporosis. Coping may require a team effort involving family and your health care team. Above all, it requires your commitment.

Practice good posture

People who have osteoporosis live with greater risk of injury from movements that involve twisting, lifting, carrying or bending. But being cautious doesn't mean that you should stop being active.

You can take steps to increase your safety and protect yourself from fractures and falls. Learning to sit, stand and move using good posture and body mechanics makes it easier to function in your daily routine.

Poor posture increases strain on your muscles and bones, causes fatigue and makes you more prone to injury. Poor posture can complicate osteoporosis. Throughout the day, including when you exercise, try to maintain good posture. By making sure you're moving safely, you can accomplish many of the tasks you set out to do.

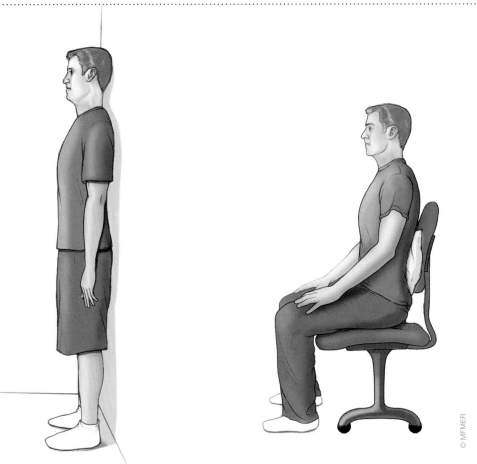

Good standing posture Head is erect with chin tucked in, chest held high, shoulders relaxed, hips level, knees straight but not locked, feet parallel.

Good sitting posture Spine and head are erect, back and legs at a 90-degree angle, natural curves of the back maintained.

Are you standing tall?

One way to correct your standing posture is with the wall test. Stand with the back of your head, shoulder blades and buttocks against a wall and your heels 2 to 4 inches from the wall.

Check the curve of your lower spine by placing your flattened hand behind the small of your back. You should be able to fit your hand snugly between your lower back and the wall. If you can fit more than a hand's thickness between your lower back and the wall, adjust your pelvis to decrease the space.

If you have difficulty placing your hand between your lower back and the wall, increase the space to attain a good posture.

Move safely

For people with osteoporosis, even mild strains and pressure can cause a fracture, so it's important to know what movements to avoid. Try to avoid bending forward, especially during activities that involve lifting or reaching. Also avoid excessive twisting of the spine. Here are some tips that can help you improve your posture:

- Think tall when you stand. Keep your stomach muscles tight.
- Stand with your weight on both of your feet.
- Wear comfortable shoes without high heels.

- When standing in one place, put one foot up on a stool or chair rung and periodically switch to the other foot.
- Don't carry a shoulder bag that weighs more than 2 pounds.
- Sit in a straight-back chair with your back supported.
- When you're in a seated position, the chair seat should be high enough so that your thighs rest horizontally on the seat and your feet are flat on the floor.
- When sitting for long periods, occasionally elevate your legs by placing your feet on a footstool. Also change positions to shift your weight. If possible, get up and move around every half-hour or so.

- When seated in bucket seats or soft chairs, use a thick rolled-up towel or pillow to support your lower back.

Coughing and sneezing

The force of a cough or sneeze can cause you to jerk forward suddenly. If your bones are weak, this could result in a compression fracture. To avoid such injury, get in the habit of placing your hand behind your back or on your thigh for support.

Working and lifting

Always strive to use good posture and body mechanics as you go about your daily activities. And ask yourself if there are new and more efficient ways to perform common activities. Remember, you don't necessarily have to do things a certain way simply because that's the way you've always done them.

Avoid movements such as reaching, bending, twisting, or using short, choppy motions, which can be dangerous for someone with osteoporosis. If you have to lift or push or pull something, use proper technique.

Sleeping

How you sleep is important, too. When lying down, you want to maintain your spine's normal curvature and avoid positions that can aggravate your back. On the opposite page are examples of sleep positions that can help prevent a fracture. Remember when on your back, don't lift your head and upper back to sit up in bed or get out of bed. Roll to your side first and then sit up.

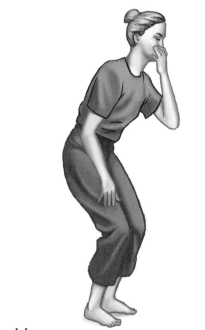

Coughing

A hand on the thigh helps support your back from the force of a sneeze.

Sleeping

Sleep on your side with your thighs somewhat drawn up toward your chest. Place a pillow between your legs.

If you sleep on your back, support your knees and neck with pillows.

Sleep on your stomach only if a pillow cushions your abdomen.

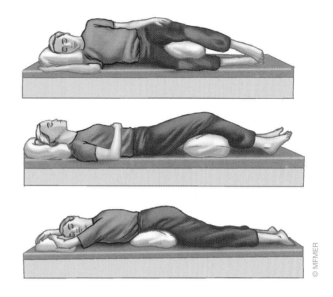

© MFMER

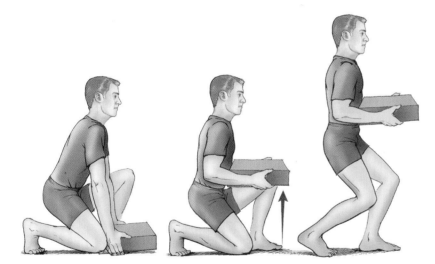

Lifting

Lifting objects, even those that are lightweight, can put stress on your spine. To lift properly:

- Keep your feet about shoulder-width apart and maintain the normal curve of your spine. Place one foot forward, and lower your body down to one knee by bending at the hips and knees, keeping your body weight on the balls of your feet.

- Kneel close to the object you're about to lift. If the object is heavy, lift it first to your bent knee.

- Grasping the object, rise from the floor by using your leg muscles. Gently breathe in while straightening up. Don't hold your breath.

- Carry the object close to your body at about waist level. If possible, place your forearms under the object. Turn by pivoting your feet. Don't twist at your waist.

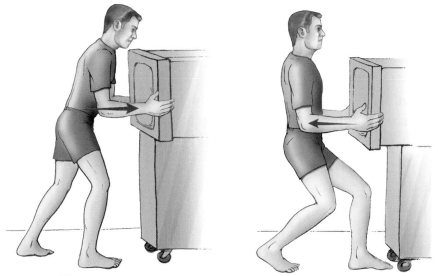

Pushing and pulling

When moving objects, you want to minimize the strain that you put on your back. Whenever possible, push rather than pull.

- Bend your knees so that your arms are level with the object. Don't bend forward at the waist.
- Maintain the normal curve of your spine and walk forward or backward, using your body weight to push or pull the object.

Using long-handled objects

The movements of raking, sweeping, mopping and vacuuming can put undue stress on your spine. To reduce this stress:

- Stand with one foot forward. Use a rocking motion to shift your body weight to your forward foot. To pull back, shift your weight to your back foot.
- Use arm and leg movements instead of back movements.
- Avoid overreaching, twisting and choppy motions. Use long, smooth strokes.

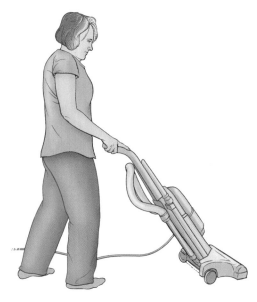

Safety tips for common daily tasks

As you perform daily chores, keep these suggestions in mind:

- If you're sweeping, use a long-handled dustpan.
- Use casters under your furniture to make moving it easier.
- An upright vacuum requires you to stoop less. Self-propelled vacuums also are easier to use.
- For mopping, fill the pail half full and lower it to the floor using both hands. Finish filling the pail with a smaller container. After mopping, empty the pail halfway using the container, then lift the bucket and dump the water down the drain.
- When changing bedding, avoid using fitted sheets unless you have a single bed or a lightweight mattress. You can tuck in the corners of a flat sheet using an open hand. If you must lift the mattress, get help.
- Carry a laundry basket that's only half full or use a basket on wheels. Be sure you can see the floor when you're walking with the basket, especially when you're on the stairs.
- Use an ironing board that's at the correct height for you. Have a clothes rack nearby to hang your ironed clothes on. And when you sort clothing, do so at a table or counter that doesn't require you to hunch forward while working.
- Drive up to the parcel pickup for your groceries or have your groceries delivered. Avoid carrying them yourself if possible, even if they seem lightweight.

Boost your emotional health

Having osteoporosis may stir a wide range of emotions. And the more severe your condition, the more intense your emotions are likely to be. When you first learn you have the disease, you may feel shock, disbelief or anger. If you've fractured a bone, you may feel helpless. Anxiety and depression also are common responses.

Negative emotions are a natural and understandable reaction to a chronic illness, but such emotions don't have to get the best of you. For many people, the first step is admitting that their negative feelings exist. This can be tough in a culture that so frequently praises the optimist and criticizes the complainer.

Fear and anxiety

"What happens if I fracture a bone?" This is one of the most common fears among people with osteoporosis. You may worry that a fracture could lead to the loss of your independence and require you to depend more on others. You may feel anxious if you can't live up to your own or others' expectations. This may be especially true if your condition limits your ability to cook, clean or care for yourself.

Fear of fracture often leads a person to limit his or her activities. Unfortunately, this can set off a vicious cycle: A more sedentary lifestyle leads to decreased physical conditioning, making you more susceptible to falls, which in turn makes you all the more reluctant to be active. Lack of activity can also lead to apathy, isolation and depression.

Depression

Depression is two to three times more common in individuals with a chronic illness compared with the general population. If your osteoporosis is keeping you from performing daily tasks or is causing you pain because of a fracture, you could be at risk of depression. Anxiety, reduced activity and changes in your physical appearance also may contribute to depression.

Depression can manifest itself in a variety of ways that you may not always recognize:

- Sleep problems
- Changes in appetite
- Loss of interest or pleasure in most activities

Controlling stress

No one is immune from stress, but a chronic condition such as osteoporosis can ratchet up your stress level. Sometimes simply becoming aware of the causes can make stress easier to deal with. Aim for a healthy balance of activities in your day — time for work, physical activity, socializing, relaxation and rest. These stress-relieving tactics may help:

Organize your day
An organized day can help you feel more in control of your life. You might start by getting out of bed 15 minutes earlier to ease the morning rush. Keep a written schedule of your daily activities so that you don't run into conflicts or last-minute panics to get to an appointment.

Plan before you act
Before you begin a task, gather all of the items you need. For example, keep cleaning supplies in one bucket to avoid multiple trips up and down the stairs. Or list the items you need before shopping, to avoid a second trip.

Keep commonly used items accessible
Organize your living space and work space so that the items you use frequently are close at hand. For example, keep your wrenches and screwdrivers on a pegboard above the workbench. Keep frequently used files on your desk.

Break apart lengthy tasks
Avoid spending too much time on one activity. Instead of spending all day planting your garden, spend one or two hours a day in the garden over three or four days.

Work at a moderate pace
Instead of rushing to complete a task, take your time and work at a comfortable speed.

- Irritability and mood swings
- Restlessness
- Feelings of hopelessness, worthlessness or guilt
- Extreme fatigue or loss of energy
- Decreased concentration, attention and memory

If you think you might be depressed, talk to your doctor or another medical professional. It's important to get treatment because untreated depression can raise your risk of other health problems. With treatment, most people who have depression show improvement, often in a matter of weeks. Treatment may include medication, psychotherapy or both.

Anger

It's natural to become angry when you're confronting a chronic illness, pain or disability. But it's unhealthy to stay angry, bottle up your feelings or express them through explosive outbursts.

Mismanaged anger, whether it's short term and intense or lingering and subdued, can lead to headaches, backaches, high blood pressure and other health problems. Anger also increases muscle tension, making it difficult to

relax. Your goal is not to abolish anger but to find healthier ways of dealing with it.

Self-esteem

Osteoporosis can deliver a blow to your self-esteem. If multiple fractures prevent you from doing your job at work, pursuing a hobby or doing household chores, you might feel less competent. This can send your self-esteem spiraling downward.

You may also be bothered by physical changes, such as a stooped posture, loss of height or protrusion of your abdomen. You may see yourself as somehow deformed.

The physical changes that occur with osteoporosis can be especially challenging in a society that so highly values youthful beauty and vigor. Under normal circumstances, these ideals are hard enough to fulfill. With fractures from osteoporosis, meeting expectations becomes even more elusive.

Coping strategies

Research shows that people diagnosed with osteoporosis can improve their

Looking good

Feeling good about how you look is closely tied to self-esteem. But finding nice-looking clothes that fit well can be challenging for some people with osteoporosis. Compression fractures of your vertebrae may cause you to lose height and develop a curved back or a protruding abdomen. Blouses and shirts may feel too tight, skirts and pants may ride too high, and dresses may appear too short in the back and too long in the front.

If you can sew, try modifying clothing patterns or tailoring store-bought clothes. Otherwise, consider the following suggestions from when buying clothing:

- Think loose. Look for blouses or shirts with loosefitting sleeves, for example, dolman or raglan sleeves.
- Buy clothes a size larger than you usually buy. A snug fit can draw attention to bumps and bulges you may want to go unnoticed.
- Choose straight-sided jackets, blazers, shirts and dresses. Go for a boxy, unstructured look. Try blouses or jackets with shoulder pads.
- Avoid clothes that accentuate the waistline. To minimize the abdomen, wear dresses with dropped waistlines.
- Keep your wardrobe simple for ease of getting your clothes on and off, and use accessories such as scarves or hats to jazz up your look.
- Experiment with different types of bras, such as front-closure bras, sports bras or those with criss-cross straps, to find one that fits well and is comfortable.

emotional well-being by being actively involved in their health management. The following strategies can help you reduce stress, anxiety and depression and boost your self-esteem.

Educate yourself

The more you know about osteoporosis, the less abstract and threatening it will seem. Fear of the unknown can cause anxiety. Understanding can calm fear. If you're afraid of falling, for example, you can minimize the risks by learning how to move safely. You'll also know that doing no activity only makes you less fit and more prone to falls.

Exercise

Research shows that regular exercise reduces the symptoms of anxiety and plays a role in treating mild to moderate depression. Exercise also promotes a better self-image and raises self-esteem. For more information about physical activity and osteoporosis, see Chapter 9.

Learn to relax

Relaxation helps to counteract stress. Relaxation can also help you cope with daily demands and remain energetic and productive. Many techniques promote relaxation, including deep breathing, progressive muscle relaxation, meditation, biofeedback, hypnosis and guided imagery. It may be helpful to learn about the various relaxation techniques from a physical therapist.

Practice positive thinking

A coping technique that many people find effective is positive self-talk. Self-talk is the endless stream of thoughts that automatically run through your head every day. These thoughts may be positive or negative.

With practice you can learn to recognize negative thoughts and replace them with positive ones. For example, if your negative thought is, "I can't do things the way I used to — I'm useless," you can replace it with a positive thought such as, "I can do much of what I want to do. As long as I don't overdo it, I can still be active." Over time, positive self-talk will become more automatic.

Manage your anger

Learn to identify what triggers your anger and recognize the warning signs. When you find yourself becoming angry, take a short timeout. Remember that you have a choice in how to respond to situations. Look for ways to release strong emotions, such as writing, listening to music, gardening or painting.

Bolster your social network

Does your social network need a boost? Consider these tips:

- Make it a point to answer all phone calls, text messages, emails and letters from family and friends.
- Accept invitations to social events.
- Take the initiative and invite someone to join in an activity.
- Become more involved in community organizations, neighborhood events and family get-togethers.
- At local gatherings, strike up a conversation when the opportunity arises.
- Join a group exercise class that's safe for someone with osteoporosis. Your doctor can advise what's appropriate.
- Set aside any past differences with friends and approach each relationship with a clean slate.

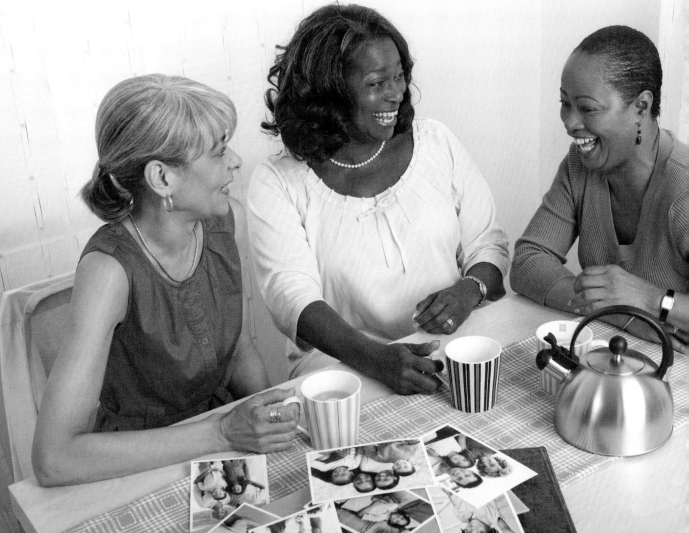

Many of these coping strategies will have a positive effect on your self-esteem. Here are other ideas for building a strong sense of self-worth:

- Structure your day with goals that you can achieve. When the day is done, you'll feel a sense of accomplishment.
- Seek emotional support. Reach out to family and friends. Confer with a counselor, religious advisor or a mental health professional.
- Help someone else. It reminds you that your life makes a difference.
- Treat yourself to something you enjoy, such as music, a book, a movie or going out with a friend.

Maintain social connections

For many people a satisfying social life is the key to feeling good mentally and physically. Social ties give you a sense of purpose in life. And staying connected is good for your health.

Studies show that people with strong social support recover from illness better than do people who face illness alone. Family and friends help you recover from any injury, including a fracture. Social contact also motivates you to be more involved in living.

Social consequences of osteoporosis

Osteoporosis can affect your relationships with family and friends in a number of ways.

Most of us define ourselves to some extent by the social positions we hold, such as parent, spouse, colleague or manager. Even mild osteoporosis can change these relationships. You may become more dependent on your spouse or adult children. You may lose a sense of shared effort and contribution within the family or at work. You may not be able to reciprocate friends' good will and intentions.

Depending on the severity of your condition or your risk of fracture, you may have to let go of some or all of your job and household responsibilities.

People with severe osteoporosis may withdraw socially because of chronic pain or fear of fractures. If you suffer from chronic pain, riding in a car, sitting in a hard chair, standing or walking can quickly become uncomfortable.

To avoid the pain, you may stop taking part in some of your customary activities, such as attending religious services, playing cards, going to movies and traveling.

Fear of falling down also can result in social isolation. You may avoid going out in public — especially to crowded places — because you worry about being pushed or stumbling. You may find it difficult to shop at grocery stores or make visits to the mall because lifting and carrying bags can be difficult.

Reaching out

Many of us are used to being quite independent. So it may seem embarrassing to ask others for help, especially with tasks you've done all of your life. But this is a time to put your safety above your independence.

Although relying on others might seem unnatural at first, this increased reliance can actually help you manage your physical health and stay independent. For example, by asking someone to help you with day-to-day tasks such as shopping and housework that require lifting, you reduce the risk of fracture. It's not a sign of weakness to ask for assistance when you need it.

It's true that relationships can sometimes be as much a source of stress as support. Your loved ones may not understand everything that you're going through emotionally, but they're likely eager to help you adjust. Family and friends can provide encouragement, offer gentle but helpful feedback and lend a hand when you need it. Remember, good relationships require patience, compromise and acceptance. Your family and friends will need to accept your needs just as you must learn to accept theirs.

Joining a support group

It can be discouraging if you feel that no one else understands exactly what you're going through. But there are people who understand, primarily because they're going through it themselves. Support groups, or self-help groups, bring together people who share common concerns. Even if your family is sympathetic, sometimes it's helpful and reassuring to talk with others in a similar situation.

A support group can give you a sense of belonging. It can provide you a place to express your feelings and fears and to exchange experiences. It also offers an opportunity to meet new friends.

Support groups may vary in format and size, but they're all based on peer support. Meetings are usually held in a library, hospital or community center. Many groups are sponsored by a hospital or a clinic or led by a health professional.

The National Osteoporosis Foundation has developed a national network of affiliated support groups. To find an osteoporosis support group in your area, ask your doctor or contact the National Osteoporosis Foundation (see page 237).

Chapter 14

Recovering from a fracture

You didn't plan on spending the next six months recovering from hip surgery. Then again, you didn't plan on slipping in the bathtub and breaking your hip either. And now here you are, using a walker to move around the house. You need help doing tasks such as the laundry and making dinner. You can't get out to see friends like you used to. You feel like you'll never be your old self again.

It's true that recuperating from a broken bone, particularly an osteoporotic fracture, can be painful, frustrating and time-consuming. But many people do regain their former abilities and a semblance of their former life. In general, the healthier you are and the more positive your attitude, the better equipped you are for recovery from a fracture.

In this chapter you'll learn how bone heals and restores itself after breaking. The discussion also includes forms of treatment for the most common osteoporotic fractures — those of the spine, hip and wrist. In addition, the chapter examines ways to manage chronic pain, which can accompany a fracture. Learning about the fracture you may have and the treatment that's available can help hasten your recovery and get you active again.

Your recovery

How well you recover from a broken bone depends in part on the location and severity of the fracture. In many instances, prompt medical attention combined with the body's natural healing process will lead to fracture repair within several months. For example, a wrist fracture will usually heal if you wear a cast and an arm sling until your wrist is stable enough to bear weight again.

But it's not always quite that simple. Additional support may be needed for severe breaks, such as hip fractures, which generally require surgery. Other fractures, such as vertebral fractures, can cause chronic pain after the bone is healed and may require a different therapeutic approach.

You'll find that each fracture requires its own course of treatment. In addition to taking steps to heal your broken bone, you may also begin receiving treatment for osteoporosis, if you haven't already done so.

But the recovery process doesn't necessarily end once the bone is healed. You may need ongoing therapy to regain most of your former strength and mobility. In addition, you may need to take steps to prevent other fractures. This often involves diet, exercise and other lifestyle changes, in addition to the use of medication.

We begin this chapter with a look at the process of bone healing.

How bone heals

As mentioned earlier, your bones are continuously renewing themselves in a process called remodeling. Cells called osteoclasts tear down, or resorb, old or damaged bone while cells called osteoblasts build new bone. This continual cycle is the basis of fracture healing. In fact, bone is the only solid tissue in your body that can replace itself. Other tissue injuries, such as a skin wound, heal with the formation of a different, fibrous tissue that leaves a scar.

Self-repair of a bone fracture can be described in phases:

Phase 1
When a bone breaks, it bleeds like any other tissue in the body. A blood clot forms that seals off damaged blood vessels near the break. Molecules in the blood clot are thought to signal specialized cells to help with the repair process. Meanwhile, osteoclasts begin removing damaged bone and tissue. Phase 1 generally takes about two weeks.

Phase 2
Over the next four weeks or so, the bone begins to regenerate with the help of osteoblasts. A soft callus that's made of collagen, the structural framework of bone, forms at the site of the break.

Phase 3

The work of the osteoblasts continues as a mesh of spongy bone develops. This creates an internal splint linking the fractured bone ends.

Phase 4

Within about six to 12 weeks, denser, harder bone replaces spongy bone. Newly deposited minerals in the collagen bind together and harden, resulting in greater bone strength. At this point, the fracture may be considered healed, although remodeling continues to strengthen the bone.

Throughout this process, the fractured bone must be correctly aligned to allow for proper healing. Problems usually arise when the ends of the fractured bone aren't aligned or they can't be immobilized. In such instances, surgery or another medical procedure may be necessary to reposition the bone ends and stabilize the fracture so that the bone will heal properly.

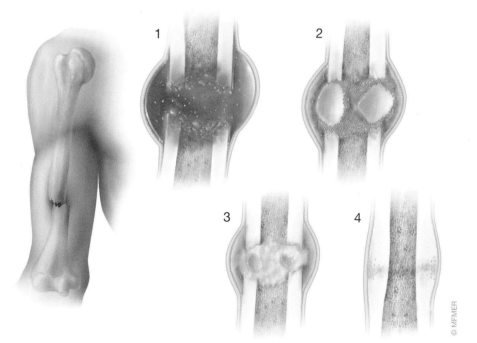

How a broken bone heals After a break, a blood clot forms, sealing off damaged blood vessels between the ends of the broken bones (1). A soft callus develops as the bone begins to regenerate (2). Osteoblasts help to build a mesh of spongy bone, creating an internal splint that links the fractured bone ends (3). With the deposit of calcium and other minerals, this mesh develops into denser bone (4).

Vertebral fractures

When the mineral density of your bones decreases, the vertebrae that make up your spinal column begin to weaken. Eventually, some vertebrae can lose most of their mineral content, leaving them unstable. The impact to bone that occurs from falling down — or even from twisting your torso improperly — can result in a compression fracture. So can lifting a load that's too heavy for your vertebrae to bear. The bone literally collapses and falls in on itself.

While some compression fractures produce no symptoms, others can cause a sudden, sharp pain or pain that's chronic and persistent.

Typically, vertebral fractures are treated with pain relievers, bed rest, braces worn around the midsection and physical therapy. Compression fractures usually heal within two to four months, and acute pain gradually recedes during this period.

Sometimes, however, the pain may persist and isn't relieved by conventional methods. In these instances, surgical procedures may be considered for treatment of fractures that cause chronic, unrelieved pain.

Pain relievers

Nonprescription pain medications often help minimize your discomfort, particularly at the start of the recovery period. Commonly used nonprescription pain relievers include aspirin, acetaminophen (Tylenol, others), ibuprofen (Advil, Motrin IB, others) and naproxen sodium (Aleve, others).

Long-term use of these medications typically isn't recommended because of the distressing side effects they can cause, such as gastrointestinal bleeding, stomach upset, dizziness, bloating and abdominal pain. Kidney problems also can occur if this type of medication is taken regularly for a lengthy amount of time.

Stronger prescription medications, such as those that contain codeine, are available for severe pain. However, prescription medications may cause constipation, which can be particularly distressing, along with other side effects. Long-term use can also lead to tolerance for the medications. When this happens, larger dosages are required to alleviate the pain.

Bed rest

Acute pain from a compression fracture will usually diminish after a couple of days of bed rest. A firm mattress provides better support for your spine than does a soft one. Although rest is essential to alleviate the initial pain, staying in bed for more than a few days generally isn't good. Doing so may weaken your back and aggravate bone loss.

Therefore, it's important to start moving as soon as you can, alternating periods of rest with activity. Physical activity can strengthen the muscles in your back and abdomen and improve support for your spine.

Bracing

If the pain persists following several days of bed rest, your doctor may recommend that you use a brace to help support your back. Back braces are generally worn for short periods of time, such as when doing an activity that may strain the back. Wearing a brace for too long can actually be counterproductive. With a brace, your back doesn't work to support itself, causing your back muscles and abdominal muscles to weaken.

Back braces are generally available at pharmacies and medical supply stores. There are many styles to choose from. Your doctor or a physical therapist can advise you on the best choice.

Exercise

Exercise can strengthen your back muscles, help you maintain good posture, slow bone loss and improve your overall fitness, all of which can help prevent fractures. Your doctor or a physical therapist can help you design a safe exercise routine that provides you with these benefits while minimizing the risk of fractures during exercise. An exercise program usually includes the following:

Weight-bearing exercises
These are activities you do on your feet with your bones supporting your weight, such as walking.

Resistance exercises
These are activities that apply force on specific muscles and bones, for example, through the use of weights.

Back-strengthening exercises
These activities help you maintain or improve your posture, which helps avoid more fractures.

Always be sure to consult your doctor or physical therapist before beginning an exercise program, as some activities or movements can increase the pain from compression fractures or even cause more fractures.

Vertebroplasty

Vertebroplasty is a surgical procedure that uses an X-ray-guided needle to inject acrylic bone cement into fractured and collapsed vertebrae. The cement hardens over a few hours, sealing and stabilizing the fractures and relieving pain. The procedure generally takes from one to two hours.

Vertebroplasty is generally used in individuals with unstable vertebral fractures or severe pain, but there are concerns as to its effectiveness. A 2011 report looked at the results of two multi-centered, randomized controlled trials of vertebroplasty — one conducted in the United States, the other based in Australia. Results from the trials failed to show an advantage among individuals who received vertebroplasty compared with those who underwent a fake procedure (placebo group).

The report doesn't totally discount the effectiveness of vertebroplasty — there are other studies that tout the procedure's benefits — but it does point to the need for additional research involving a greater number of people to bring about more definitive results.

Complications of the procedure are relatively few. During the hardening process, the cement generates heat that threatens nerve endings within the spine. This may cause temporary discomfort, but may also provide some pain relief.

One of the main concerns surrounding vertebroplasty is leakage of the cement into surrounding tissues as it's being injected. During test studies, the leakage generally had no side effects, although in a few incidents it led to compressed nerves and increased pain.

Kyphoplasty

Kyphoplasty is a surgical procedure similar to vertebroplasty that involves the use of a balloon-tipped needle. After the needle is inserted into the vertebra, the balloon is inflated to create a space for the cement to be injected. In most cases, this action not only strengthens the vertebra but also may expand the collapsed vertebral body.

Kyphoplasty is reported to provide pain relief, and serious complications are uncommon. But, again, health experts caution that more research is necessary to determine all of the procedure's risks and benefits, as well as its effectiveness.

Hip fractures

A hip fracture is a serious injury, particularly if you're older, and its complications can be life-threatening. Most hip fractures occur in people older than 65, with the risk increasing most rapidly after age 80.

A hip fracture almost always requires surgical repair or replacement, followed by physical therapy. Doctors may turn to nonsurgical alternatives, such as traction, only if you have a serious illness that makes surgery too risky. The type of surgery you have generally depends on where the bone is broken, the severity of the fracture and your age.

Femoral neck fractures

The long bone of your thigh (femur) is connected to the pelvis at your hip, which is a ball-and-socket joint. A narrow section of the femur just below the joint, known as the femoral neck, is a common location for a hip fracture (see page 40). Doctors repair the fracture by one of three methods:

Internal fixation
Surgeons may insert metal screws into the bone to hold it together while the fracture heals. In some cases, screws are attached to a metal plate that runs down alongside the femur.

Partial hip replacement
If the ends of the broken bone aren't properly aligned or they've been damaged, your doctor may remove the head and neck of the femur and install a metal replacement (prosthesis).

Total hip replacement
A total hip replacement involves replacing both your upper femur and the socket in your pelvic bone with prostheses. Total hip replacement may be a good option if arthritis or a prior injury has damaged your joint, affecting its function even before the fracture.

Intertrochanteric region fractures

The intertrochanteric region is the part of a femur adjacent to the femoral neck.

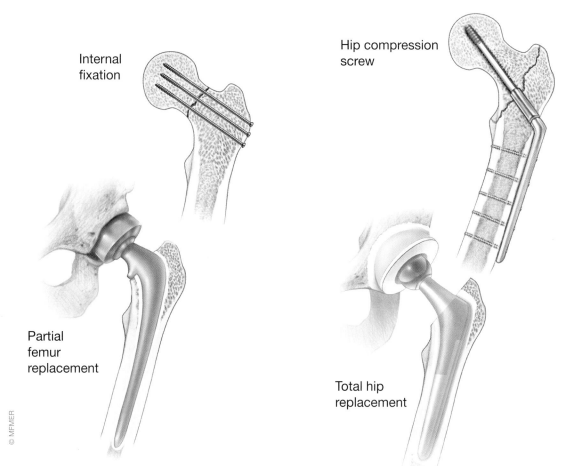

Internal fixation

Hip compression screw

Partial femur replacement

Total hip replacement

© MFMER

Treatment options for a hip fracture For a fracture in the femoral neck, internal fixation, partial femur replacement or a total hip replacement may be used. A hip compression screw may be used for a fracture in the intertrochanteric region.

To repair a fracture in this area, a surgeon usually inserts a long metal screw, known as a hip compression screw, through the fracture to rejoin the broken bone. The screw is attached to a plate that runs partially down the length of the femur. The plate is attached to the femur with smaller screws to keep the bone stable. As the bone heals, the compression screw allows the edges to grow together.

General concerns

When you have hip surgery, you'll either undergo general anesthesia or local anesthesia. If all or part of the joint is removed, the prosthesis is often secured with bone cement — the same type that's used in vertebroplasty and kyphoplasty. It takes only a few hours for the cement to harden and the hip prosthesis to be firmly in place.

Sometimes a different type of prosthesis is used that allows the bone itself to grow into the device and keep it in place. This usually requires a longer recovery period because the bone needs time to grow. A hybrid prosthesis involves cementing part of the device (usually the socket) and leaving the other part uncemented (usually the femoral neck).

Artificial hip joints generally can function well for 20 years or more, but eventually the prosthesis may loosen, necessitating another operation. Older adults are more likely to receive a partial or total hip replacement because they tend to put less strain on an artificial joint than younger people do. Among younger individuals, use of internal fixation to repair a fractured hip is more common, however the procedure can be used to repair fractures in people of any age so long as the broken bones are well-aligned.

If the hip is infected or there's a skin disorder around the hip, a surgeon will likely wait until the condition improves before doing the operation. Before surgery you'll probably go through an extensive evaluation to check your medical history, the extent of damage to your hip and your current health. Your doctor likely will also discuss the potential risks and benefits of having hip surgery in your specific case.

At the hospital

Hip surgery usually requires a few days to a week in the hospital, depending on how well you recover from the operation. Hospital staff will try to get you up and moving as soon as possible.

A serious complication of hip surgery is the formation of blood clots in the veins of your thighs and calves. A blood clot may break free and travel to your lungs, causing a pulmonary embolism that can be fatal in a matter of hours. Hospital staff will closely monitor your condition to prevent this from happening.

It's important to begin gentle activity immediately after surgery. This may include slowly moving your foot up and down or rotating your ankle as you lie in bed. A physical therapist can show you how to do specific exercises. Although these activities might feel uncomfortable at first, they can lessen pain, prevent blood clot formation and improve hip movement.

You'll likely continue these exercises after you go home. In addition, your doctor may prescribe blood-thinning medications for several weeks or months after the procedure to prevent clot formation, as well as antibiotics to prevent infections. Some older adults, particularly those who live alone, may enter a rehabilitation center for a period of time after surgery to receive physical therapy and assistance during their recovery.

At home

Before you go home, or even before you enter the hospital for surgery, it may be a good idea to have your home rearranged to be more conducive to recovery. This involves clearing pathways so that you can freely use a walker and making sure that you have a firm, high-seated chair available that you can use.

In addition, set up a personal recovery area with everything you need at your fingertips, such as eyeglasses, reading material, medications, a phone, a remote control, a computer or tablet, a wastebasket, and water to drink.

You contribute much to your own rehabilitation. Your participation in the recovery process often determines the procedure's success. Here are a number of factors to keep in mind:

- Keep the incision clean and dry. Stitches are generally removed two to three weeks after surgery. Until then take sponge baths instead of showers or full baths.
- Swelling is a normal reaction during the first few months after surgery. To counteract the swelling, elevate your leg and place an ice pack on your hip for several minutes at a time. Avoid placing ice directly on your skin by wrapping the pack in a washcloth or dish towel.
- Contact your doctor immediately if you think you're developing a blood clot or infection. Signs and symptoms of a blood clot include pain, redness or tenderness in your calf, and new swelling in your leg or foot. Signs and symptoms of an infection include redness or swelling around the incision, wound drainage, persistent high fever, chills and increasing hip pain.
- Care must be taken not to dislocate the prosthesis. Don't cross your legs, whether sitting, standing or lying down. Keep your knees below the level of your hips. Sit on a cush-

ion to keep your hips higher than your knees. Avoid bending at the waist. When sleeping, place a pillow between your knees to keep your hip properly aligned.

- Because bacteria can enter your bloodstream during dental procedures, it's important to let your dentist know that you've had a hip replacement. Your dentist may recommend that you take antibiotics before dental work to help prevent bacteria buildup and an infection.
- It's important to stay active. Get up and move around at least once an hour during the day. If you have a cemented or hybrid prosthesis, you can usually put some weight on your leg right away, but you'll need to use a walker for a while to allow the joint to heal properly. If you have a cementless prosthesis, your surgeon will probably ask you not to put any weight on the leg for the first six weeks, to give your bones time to grow into the prosthesis.
- Don't overdo your activities. The key is to be active and exercise at a level that's comfortable for you. Walking is usually safe, and swimming, an exercise that's easy on your joints, is recommended after your incision has healed.
- A healthy diet is important. If you were watching your weight before surgery, continue doing so because excess weight can place unnecessary stress on your hip joint.

Most people return to their normal activities. But it generally doesn't happen immediately. A healthy recovery requires not only a willingness to do what your doctor or physical therapist prescribes but also consistency in actually doing it, such as performing prescribed exercises each day.

Wrist fractures

Compared with vertebral and hip fractures, wrist fractures are usually simpler to treat. Most osteoporotic wrist fractures — about 90 percent — are clean breaks of the radial bone in the forearm just above the wrist joint. This break is known as a Colles' fracture. These types of fractures typically heal well, resulting in full use of the hand and wrist.

Some wrist fractures, however, can be complex. If the broken ends of bone shift apart by less than a tenth of an inch, the fracture is considered displaced. Before the bone is allowed to heal, the bone must be realigned. If a bone splinters into numerous

When treatment doesn't prevent a fracture

A person with osteoporosis who is taking medication to prevent fractures might still experience a fracture. In most cases, this occurs because osteoporosis medications — at best — prevent about only 70 percent of fractures. In addition, some osteoporosis medications are more effective in preventing fractures than are others. And while all osteoporosis medications help prevent spinal fractures, not all medications prevent hip, wrist or other fractures. Your doctor will select the right type of medication for you, based on your initial bone density test report and your risk of future fractures.

So, what do you do if you experience a fracture while receiving treatment for osteoporosis? It's likely that your doctor will review your situation to make sure that you're taking the medication correctly. Because some individuals don't absorb the medication properly, your doctor may also order tests to rule this out as a possible cause for your fracture. Depending on when you had your last bone density test, your doctor may have you take another test to see if your bone density has improved, remained stable or decreased. If you're receiving treatment, your bone density should remain stable or improve. If your bone density decreases, this could be a sign that your medication isn't working.

It may also be that the cause of your bone loss is a condition neither you nor your doctor are aware of that isn't being adequately treated. This condition may produce a stronger negative effect on your bones than the positive effect of your medication. For example, your vitamin D level might be too low, such that you can't absorb calcium adequately. Your bone density may decrease because of this, despite taking your medication. To rule out an unrecognized cause, you may be asked to undergo several blood or urine tests, or both.

Even after checking for a variety of conditions, some people have no identifiable cause for their fractures. In this type of circumstance, it's likely that your doctor will continue to use the same kind of medication, and it may be that no further fractures will occur. If another fracture does occur, you may be switched to a different, more powerful drug.

pieces, the break is referred to as a comminuted fracture.

In either case, surgery may be required to reposition the pieces, and various devices may be used to hold the pieces in place as the bone heals. If the broken bone breaks the skin — what's known as an open fracture — emergency treatment is required to prevent infection.

Several methods are used to treat a fractured wrist:

Cast or splint

A cast is often the preferred method for older adults who have a simple wrist fracture with minimal displacement. A short arm cast is usually applied from below the elbow to the hand. It immobilizes the wrist bone, is less invasive than is surgery and usually has good results. After a fracture, swelling is often a problem. If so, a splint may be used for the first few days and then replaced with a cast after the swelling has gone down. Elevating your arm and icing your hand also helps to diminish the swelling.

In other cases, a long arm cast, which extends from your upper arm to your hand, is used to immobilize the whole arm and thumb. The long arm cast is later replaced with a short arm cast to allow free motion of the elbow. After

the cast is removed, your doctor may have you use a removable splint at night and between exercise sessions during the day for added support.

Internal fixation

Some complex fractures, particularly those that extend into the joint, may require internal fixation. This involves surgery in which a surgeon places metal pins, rods, plates, screws or bone grafts inside or along the fracture to hold the bone in position as it heals.

External fixation

If a fracture is severely displaced or comminuted, it may heal best with metal pins inserted through the skin into the bone on either side of the fracture. The pins are attached externally to a frame that helps hold the fracture in place. Your arm is held in a sling to help protect it and to keep the wrist elevated. An external device is usually worn for six to 12 weeks. During this time, your doctor may adjust the pins periodically to ensure the precise alignment of the bone.

Injectable bone cement

For some fractures, a bone-replacement material is used that acts as a filler, helping to restore stability to the broken bone. Bone cement used to be more commonly used for wrist and hand fractures, but the results were often unsatisfactory. It is now mainly reserved for unique cases.

Physical therapy

A frequent complication of a wrist fracture is subsequent stiffness of the wrist. To counteract this effect, your doctor or physical therapist likely will work with you to get your fingers and adjoining elbow and shoulder moving as soon as possible after the fracture has stabilized.

A common exercise is to close your fingers into a fist and then slowly fully extend them. You may be asked to do this several times an hour during the day. After the cast or fixation device is removed, you'll be given additional exercises, including resistance exercises to build bone mass. You may also receive balance and gait training to prevent further falls.

As with any form of rehabilitation, you play a vital role. Your goal is to regain function of your hand. You may accomplish this by following your doctor's instructions carefully and by consistently performing the prescribed exercises.

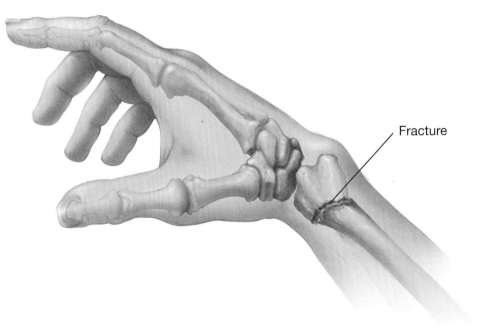

Fracture

© MFMER

Wrist fracture Wrist fractures may be treated in a number of different ways. A basic fracture is often treated with a cast. For more severe fractures, metal pins may be used to help hold the bones in place while the fracture heals.

Managing chronic pain

Although proper treatment may relieve the initial pain of an osteoporotic fracture, the recovery period following treatment also can be painful. Sometimes pain may persist after the bone has healed.

Dealing with chronic pain can be frustrating when there seems to be no immediate relief in sight. The pain can cause feelings of irritability, depression and anxiety, which only make the pain seem worse. Although no quick fixes are available, you can learn to manage your pain. Keep these two points in mind:

- **You play a central role in pain management.** If you want your life to improve, you'll need to take steps to make it happen. Only you can control your future.
- **Managing chronic pain isn't about making pain disappear.** It's about learning to keep pain at a level you can tolerate.

In dealing with chronic pain, people often turn to pain medications. These are certainly appropriate for coping with acute pain, and they can be very effective when used properly. But for many chronic pain disorders, medication often isn't the answer.

Some people take medication because they feel they need to, not because it helps. The drugs become a crutch or distraction from more-effective, safer, long-term solutions. These people are often surprised to find that stopping their medications isn't as difficult as they had anticipated. They also often find that not using medications gives them a greater sense of control over the pain and their lives.

Alternative methods for relieving pain

When medication isn't effective or it isn't recommended due to unwanted side effects, other methods can be used to help relieve chronic pain.

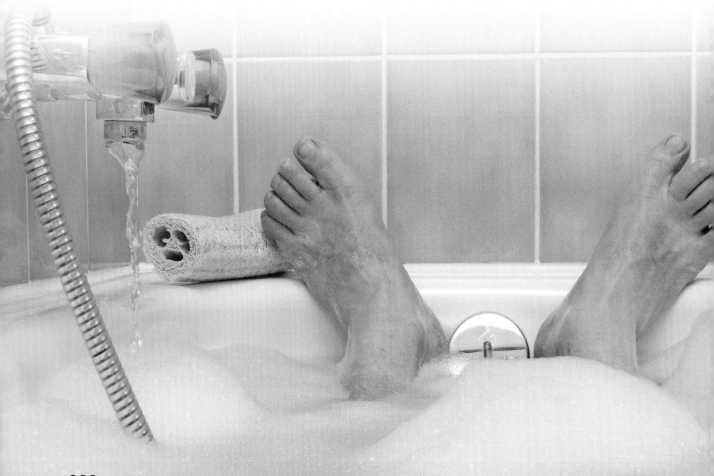

Exercise

Although rest is important for recovery and pain relief, exercise is equally vital to reducing pain, especially in the long term. Exercise causes your body to release chemicals called endorphins, which block pain signals from reaching your brain. The more endorphins you produce on your own, the less you need to rely on other forms of pain management, such as medication.

Because certain exercises shouldn't be done when you have osteoporosis, it's important to consult your doctor before beginning an exercise program. That way you'll be sure you're performing the activities that are best for you.

Ice and heat

Applying an ice pack can reduce swelling and inflammation and act as a local anesthetic. Treatment in the form of a hot water bottle, hot bath or heat lamp relaxes your muscles and helps relieve chronic pain. Remember not to directly expose your skin to extreme temperatures. Keep the ice pack or hot water bottle wrapped in a towel. Limit applications to 20 minutes at a time.

Relaxation techniques

Your physical therapist can show you certain relaxation techniques that help take your mind off pain, relax your muscles and relieve unnecessary stress. These techniques might include visualization, progressive muscle relaxation and deep breathing.

Biofeedback

The goal of biofeedback is to teach you how to control certain body responses. During a biofeedback session, a trained therapist applies electrodes and other sensors to various parts of your body. The electrodes are attached to devices that monitor your responses and give you visual or auditory feedback of your muscle tension, heart rate, blood pressure, breathing rate and skin temperature.

With this feedback you can learn to produce positive changes in body functions, such as lowering your blood pressure or raising your skin temperature. These are signs of relaxation. And remember, the more relaxed you are, the less focused you are on your pain. The biofeedback therapist may use relaxation techniques to further calm you.

Music therapy

Practitioners of music therapy claim that it can lower stress, reduce symptoms of depression and promote pain relief. With this treatment, a trained music therapist uses music and all of its facets — physical, emotional, mental, social and spiritual — to help individuals improve or maintain their health. Performing or listening to music, with guidance from a music therapist, can help relieve muscle tension and slow your breathing.

Electrical stimulation

Transcutaneous electrical nerve stimulation (TENS) may help stop pain by blocking nerve signals from reaching your brain. A physical therapist places electrodes on your skin near the area of your pain. TENS may relieve pain in your leg due to inflammation or compression of nerves in your back, but it may provide little relief for chronic back pain.

A word of caution

Certain methods of pain relief may spell trouble if you have osteoporosis. Massage, chiropractic treatment and other spinal manipulation can cause or aggravate vertebral fractures, so talk to your doctor before trying any of these.

Chapter 15

Home safety

Falls are a serious hazard for older adults, especially those with osteoporosis. According to the Centers for Disease Control and Prevention, 1 out of every 3 people in the United States age 65 years and older will fall each year. And of those who fall, 20 to 30 percent will suffer moderate to severe injuries that reduce their mobility and independence. At least 95 percent of all hip fractures result from a fall.

Among people age 65 and older, half of all falls occur at home. Therefore, it's simple logic that an action plan for osteoporosis involves minimizing your risk of falling. You may do so by organizing your home environment and work space in a way that allows you to function and move about comfortably and safely.

You may also have occasion to use what are known as assistive devices. These are items or pieces of equipment that enable you to perform routine tasks and activities safely and with minimum stress. Canes and walkers can provide support and keep you balanced as you move about. Other assistive devices eliminate dangerous movements that can lead to fracture, such as reaching above your head for something on a high shelf or bending forward to pick up something off the floor.

If you're like most people, you likely want to remain as independent as you can. Often, this means being able to live at home, keep your own schedule and organize your time as freely as anyone else. To be able to do this for as long a time as reasonably possible, some preventive action is necessary. This chapter focuses on practical measures you can take to help prevent fractures, stay active and maintain the lifestyle you want.

Staying safe indoors

It's ironic that the home — your private sanctum — statistically ranks as one of the most dangerous places you can be. But you have to remember that the average residence puts you in regular contact with electricity, heat sources, water, slick surfaces, stairs and many other physical dangers. And many people, particularly older adults, spend a major portion of each 24-hour day within the walls of their homes.

For these reasons, it's important to survey your home and look for features that could cause you to lose your balance or footing: stairs, rugs, electrical cords, step stools and locations in the home where there may be wet surfaces. The kitchen and bathroom are often among the most dangerous places in the home. Also identify high-traffic areas that combine multiple threats.

Keep in mind these general principles when inspecting your home for safety: Keep pathways clear, use proper lighting and safe seating, and organize work areas.

Keep pathways clear

Clearly, you need to watch your footing everywhere you go in your home. But pay close attention to the primary pathways within rooms, between rooms and in hallways. Keep these areas picked up and remove unnecessary clutter.

Also be alert to tight spaces and blind corners that might cause you to bump into furniture or collide with someone. Avoid loose rugs and carpeting, buckled or torn linoleum or tile, and raised thresholds — the crosspiece at the bottom of a door frame — that could catch your heel and cause a fall.

Use proper lighting

Good vision is one of the best tools you have to prevent falls. The easiest, most practical way to improve vision safety in your home is to add lighting. Be prepared to add more than just an extra lamp or two. Start by increasing

Taking steps to prevent falls

Here are some simple changes you can make in your home to prevent falls:

- Keep rooms free of clutter, especially floors.
- Keep electrical and telephone cords tucked out of the way.
- Avoid walking in socks, stockings or plush slippers. Choose comfortable, low-heeled shoes with nonskid soles.
- Be sure your carpets and rugs have skidproof backing or are tacked to the floor. Get rid of throw rugs.
- Place a phone and flashlight within reach of your bed.
- Make sure stairs are well-lit and have handrails on both sides. Cover the steps with tightly woven carpet or nonslip treads.
- Install grab bars on bathroom walls near the tub, shower and toilet. Use a rubber mat in the tub and shower.
- Use a night light in your bathroom.
- Add ceiling fixtures so that you don't have to walk into a dark room to turn on a lamp.

the wattage in the lamps you currently use. Be careful to stay within the manufacturer's recommended range for each fixture, which is marked on the device. Be aware, also, that too much light used in the wrong way can produce a blinding glare.

Areas of your home that may need the greatest lighting improvement are stairways, hallways, storage closets, storage sheds, the laundry room, the garage and locations with a change in floor height, for example, a sunken living room. Check to see that you have the highest wattage bulbs allowed in overhead lights. Installing lighting under kitchen cabinets helps brighten work areas.

Because your balance may not be as good in the dark as it is during daylight hours, place night lights in key pathways of your house. They're great for illuminating midnight trips to the bathroom and kitchen.

Ask an electrician about adding three- or four-way wall switches to your heavily used rooms. These allow you to control lights from more than one location, saving you a trip across a dark room. The technology for remote control switches has improved dramatically, as has the cost of these safety devices.

Use safe seating

Keep furniture, especially chairs, sofas and other forms of seating, in good repair. Chairs should be well-supported and not prone to tipping. Be cautious with anything on rollers or rockers. To prevent dizziness that contributes to falls, sit down or stand up slowly.

It's important that you are able to sit down or stand up easily and without unnecessary strain. Particularly after hip replacement, you'll need to keep your hips higher than your knees to prevent dislocating the new joint. Chairs or sofas that sit high with firm cushioning are generally easier to get in and out of than low, soft-cushioned seating. You may be able to adapt existing furniture with an extra foam cushion or two placed on the chair or under the sofa cushioning.

Organize work areas

Keep frequently used items within easy reach and avoid stretching for items on high shelves. If you must retrieve something high above you, use a sturdy step stool with wide steps and handrails or an assistive device known as a reacher. In the kitchen you can limit strain on your back by using front burners on your stove whenever possible and sliding, not lifting, pots in and out of the oven.

Exposure to tap water that's too hot can cause you to pull back suddenly and possibly slip and fall, especially in the bathtub. To prevent scalding from hot water, be sure the water heater thermostat isn't set too high. Clean up any spills on the floor immediately.

Assistive devices

Everyone has heard the phrase "Work smarter, not harder." If you swap the word *live* for *work*, you'll begin to understand the idea behind assistive devices. These tools for living smarter can help you with everyday tasks. Some are simple handle extensions that provide more leverage, and others are sophisticated, ergonomically designed devices.

Gadgets and gimmicks aren't for you, you say? That initial reaction is typical — even understandable. But before you associate assistive devices with wasted money or physical weakness, consider how many of them we already rely on to make our lives easier and more enjoyable.

It's unlikely, for example, that you hesitate before climbing into an automobile for a short drive to the grocery store. A car is an assistive device. The vehicle certainly helps you get from one point to another with greater speed and comfort than you would have by walking. What about the remote control that allows you to flick through television channels while seated in a comfortable chair across the room? A remote control also is an assistive device.

Assistive devices generally have a well-defined function and are easy to use, sometimes with a little practice. Whether it's something you do every day, such as putting on your shoes, or something you do once in a while, such as moving a heavy object, these devices help you achieve your goals with minimum risk to your bones. Gait aids, such as a cane or walker, allow you to put more energy into mobility and less into stability — you can walk farther, faster and more safely.

Medical supply stores, websites, catalogs, your hospital's physical therapy department and even the local hardware store are full of specifically designed items and materials that can help you with daily tasks. By using these tools, you can ease pain, add comfort, increase safety, bolster confidence, enhance ability and sustain independence.

Devices for daily needs

Assistive devices are often used to accomplish simple daily tasks. Using the right tool can facilitate almost everything you need to do or want to do at home. One of the most common and practical tools is what's known as a reacher. This device is a lightweight pole with a trigger at one end that manipulates a single grasping claw at the other end. A reacher can help you retrieve lightweight items such as a newspaper from the floor or a remote control from the coffee table without having to bend forward. The device is easily carried and can be used just about anywhere in the house.

Many such helpful devices are available for use in the bathroom. These include grab bars and folding shower seats to prevent slipping, and elevated toilets that permit easier seating. You can buy long-handled hairbrushes, combs and sponges to clean and groom yourself without having to twist or bend your torso.

In the kitchen, chances are you're already using some small electric appliances. You can expand their usefulness

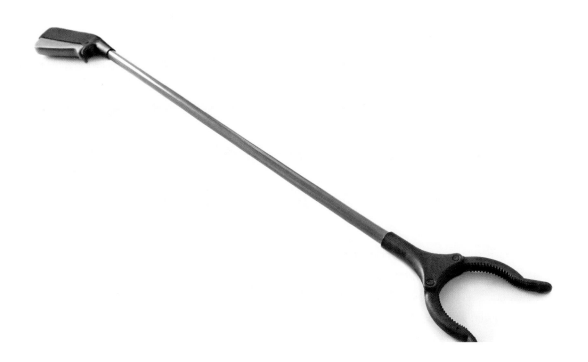

by finding new ways to adapt them to your chores. Manufacturers of appliances sometimes include tips for alternative uses. Buy a jar opener that can be mounted under a kitchen cabinet or countertop. A reacher with a squeeze-handle grasper is perfect for easy access to items on higher or lower shelves.

Devices for movement and mobility

If you've had hip surgery, you may need support as you move around the house, at least during the first few months of recovery. Multiple compression fractures of the spine that cause you to hunch forward also may require you to use a cane or walker.

According to the Department of Health and Human Services, millions of Americans use assistive devices to accommodate impairments with walking. Although they may initially seem awkward and annoying, walking aids help you get around on your own.

Walking aids include canes and walkers. Each type comes in a variety of sizes, weights and designs, so it's not always easy to select and properly use the right one.

It may be best to have your doctor or physical therapist recommend a walking aid that would be most appropriate for you. Get assistance in determining the proper size and fit, as well as the best way to use it and adapt it to your needs. It's a common mistake to choose a cane that's too long. The extra length pushes up one arm and shoulder, causing strain on certain back muscles.

Awkwardness with any new device is natural. Remember the first time you tried riding a bike or casting a fishing rod? Ease will come with practice. Here are some pointers to help you be more informed about your options.

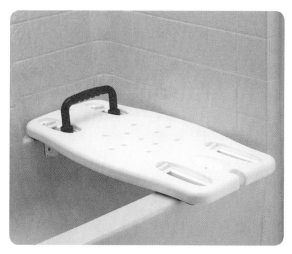

Preventing falls The bathroom is a common place for falls because of wet surfaces. A number of devices, such as the shower chair shown here, can make getting around the bathroom less risky.

Canes

Canes aren't intended to carry the full weight of your body. Rather, they provide some relief and stability by allowing you to put a third point of contact on the ground — besides your two feet.

If you need to use your cane daily, the traditional J-handle (candy-cane) style may not be your best choice. That's because with a J-handle your weight isn't centered over the cane's shaft, which puts more pressure on your hand. Instead, consider using the swan neck cane, in which the shaft absorbs more of your weight. Other handgrip styles and shapes are available. Choose the one that feels most comfortable.

Quadripod canes, which have four feet, offer greater stability than do canes with a single tip, but they can be cumbersome to use. A lightweight aluminum cane is often less of a burden than is a heavier wooden one.

To see if your cane is the right fit, stand erect with your shoes on, letting your arms hang at your sides. The top of the cane's handle should align with

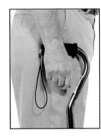

The handle of your cane should reach the crease of your wrist. When grasping the cane, your elbow should be at a 15- to 20-degree angle.

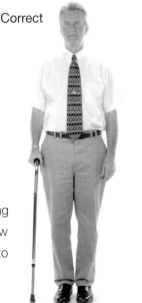

Correct

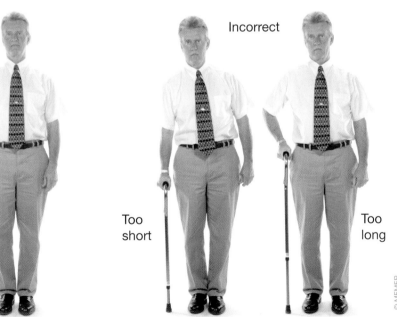

Incorrect

Too short

Too long

© MFMER

Is the height right? A proper fit for your cane is important. Canes that are the wrong height for you can cause falls as well as arm and back pain.

the crease of your wrist. When you hold the cane while standing still, your elbow should be flexed at a 15- to 20-degree angle. Wooden canes must be cut to the correct height. Adjustable canes can be lengthened or shortened to fit.

It's best to hold your cane in the hand opposite the side that needs support, regardless of which hand is your dominant or preferred hand. The cane and the affected leg should swing forward and touch the ground at the same time.

On stairs, step up with your good leg, then bring your affected leg and cane up. This way, your good leg lifts your body. Coming down the stairs, lead with your affected leg and cane, then bring your good leg down. This allows your good leg to lower your body.

Walkers

Walkers are self-standing units that provide more stability than does a cane. Some are maneuvered by lifting, and others are equipped with wheels. Some walkers are equipped with a basket or a carrying case. Walkers function best in single-level homes, and they shouldn't be used on stairs or in crowded, cluttered areas.

In general, walkers with wheels are easier to manage than walkers that you lift, unless you have thick carpet or are on rough ground. Wheeled walkers are especially important if you have balance problems. If you'll be doing any traveling, consider a walker that folds.

Because a walker disrupts your normal walking gait, you'll need a little practice. First of all, as with a cane, your walker needs to be adjusted to the correct height. When your arms are relaxed at your sides, the top of the

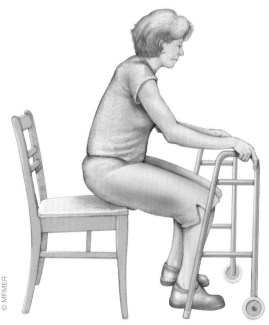

Walkers provide stability Walkers with wheels may be easier to manage than walkers that you lift. When standing up with a walker, slide toward the edge of your chair before trying to get up.

walker should align with the crease in your wrist. If your walker is adjusted correctly, you should be able to stand up straight when using it.

To walk, move the walker a comfortable arm's length from you. Don't move it too far in front, or you might fall. Then step into the walker, leading with your weak or injured leg. Don't attempt to climb stairs with a walker unless you've had training.

Grips and tips

With any walking aid, a handle that's contoured to your grip is usually easier to hold for extended periods than is a rounded handle. Wrap foam around a handle that feels too small.

The tips of walking devices come in different diameters and styles. What's important is the traction they provide with the ground. Rubber is a commonly used material because it's nonskid and easily replaced when worn out. Flat, soft tips hold the ground more securely than rounded ones do.

Never glue on the tips. You'll need to replace them as they wear out. Most pharmacies and some hardware stores carry replacement tips.

Take your time

If you're going to be using a walking aid for a while, invest some time in choosing the right style and fit for you. You can find walking aids at medical supply stores and some pharmacies. You can also order them from specialty catalogs or online.

As for cost, more expensive models aren't necessarily better at providing support than less expensive ones are. Medicare or your private insurance company may cover part or all of the cost of your walking aid if you have a written prescription from your doctor.

An open mind

Assistive devices can't do all things for all people. You can't expect a single implement to free you from issues associated with having osteoporosis or allow you to be totally independent. But assistive devices can still have a tremendous impact. It's common for people to marvel over how much easier life has become with that extra little bit of assistance, once they start using them.

To maintain your independence, keep an open mind about your physical limitations — a realistic grasp of what you can and can't do — and the tools that can help you overcome or minimize these limitations.

Whether you should use assistive devices depends on you, your doctor, or an occupational or physical therapist. Some of the tools described in this chapter may or may not be right for you. For a more customized evaluation, contact an occupational therapist.

Occupational therapists specialize in helping people deal with the effects of illness, injury or aging in their daily lives. A therapist typically can meet with you on an individual basis and make recommendations based on your specific needs. Assistive devices can be obtained from a hospital's physical therapy department, medical supply stores, specialized catalogs or Internet sites, and even local hardware stores.

The importance of attitude

All this talk about prevention and assistive devices and safe movements may leave you feeling as if life has definitely changed, and not for the better. What

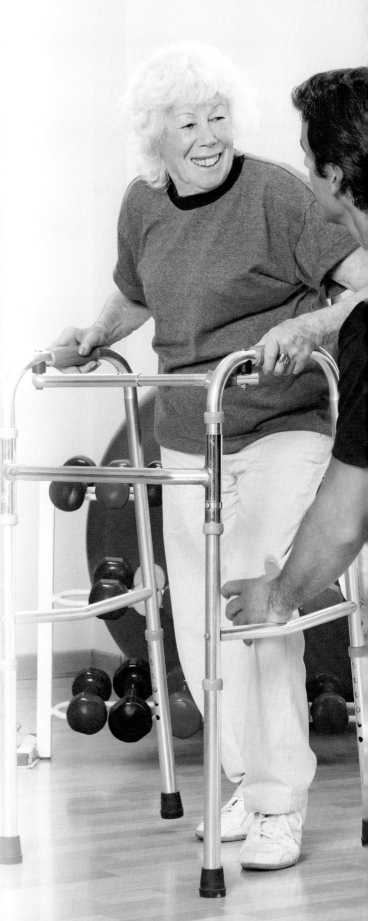

happened to the days when you moved around and did whatever you pleased without giving it a second thought? Though you've heard the following before, it still rings true: One of the constant things in life is change. How you cope with change can have a big impact on your quality of life.

Your attitude about having osteoporosis and the lifestyle adjustments you may have to make has a tremendous influence on how independent or dependent you eventually become.

For example, if you look at your cane as a sign of weakness and deterioration, you might avoid using it and end up falling and breaking a hip. But if you view your cane as a symbol of freedom and opportunity, you'll make it work for you. You'll benefit from the support and stability it provides, and you'll value the ability to move around without the aid of others.

allows you to benefit from diet, exercise, medications, good posture, and a safe environment at home or work.

Just as important to success is the support you receive from your doctor, other health care professionals, and your family and friends. All of these factors in combination can provide you with the means to prevent or treat osteoporosis and maintain a full and active life.

Taking control

It's never too late to work on maintaining or improving bone health. This book discusses many ways to approach this. A well-organized action plan suited to your needs and abilities

Additional resources

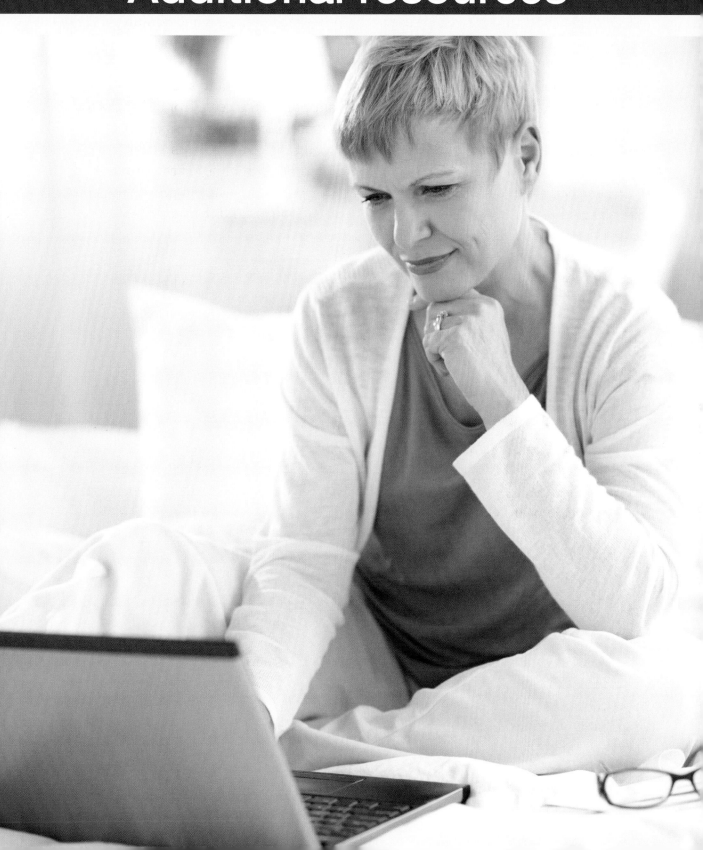

Academy of Nutrition and Dietetics
120 South Riverside Plaza, Suite 2000
Chicago, IL 60606-6995
800-877-1600
www.eatright.org

Administration for Community Living
U.S. Department of Health and Human Services
1 Massachusetts Ave., NW
Washington, DC 20201
202-357-3566
www.acl.gov

American Academy of Orthopaedic Surgeons
6300 N. River Road
Rosemont, IL 60018-4262
847-823-7186
www.aaos.org

American Academy of Physical Medicine and Rehabilitation
9700 W. Bryn Mawr Ave., Suite 200
Rosemont, IL 60018
847-737-6000
www.aapmr.org

American Association of Clinical Endocrinologists
245 Riverside Ave., Suite 200
Jacksonville, FL 32202
904-353-7878
www.aace.com

American Physical Therapy Association
1111 N. Fairfax St.
Alexandria, VA 22314-1488
800-999-2782
www.apta.org

Food and Drug Administration
U.S. Department of Health and Human Services
10903 New Hampshire Ave.
Silver Spring, MD 20993
888-463-6332
www.fda.gov

Food and Nutrition Information Center
National Agricultural Library
10301 Baltimore Ave., Room 108
Beltsville, MD 20705
301-504-5414
fnic.nal.usda.gov

HealthyWoman
National Women's Health Resource Center
157 Broad St., Suite 200
Red Bank, NJ 07701
877-986-9472
www.healthywomen.org

International Osteoporosis Foundation
9, rue Juste-Olivier
CH-1260 Nyon
Switzerland
41-22-994-0100
www.osteofound.org

Mayo Clinic Health Information
www.mayoclinic.org

National Center for Injury Prevention and Control
Centers for Disease Control and
Prevention
1600 Clifton Road
Atlanta, GA 30333
800-232-4636
www.cdc.gov/injury

National Institute for Occupational Safety and Health
Centers for Disease Control and
Prevention
1600 Clifton Road
Atlanta, GA 30333
800-232-4636
www.cdc.gov/niosh

National Institute of Arthritis and Musculoskeletal and Skin Diseases
1 AMS Circle
Bethesda, MD 20892-0001
877-226-4267
www.niams.nih.gov

National Institute on Aging
U.S. Department of Health and Human
Services
Building 31, Room 5C27
31 Center Drive, MSC 2292
Bethesda, MD 20892
800-222-2225
www.nia.nih.gov

National Osteoporosis Foundation
1150 17th St., NW, Suite 850
Washington, DC 20036
800-231-4222
nof.org

National Rehabilitation Information Center
8400 Corporate Drive, Suite 500
Landover, MD 20785
800-346-2742
www.naric.com

National Safety Council
1121 Spring Lake Drive
Itasca, IL 60143-3201
800-621-7615
www.nsc.org

NIH Osteoporosis and Related Bone Diseases — National Resource Center
National Institutes of Health (NIH)
2 AMS Circle
Bethesda, MD 20892-0001
800-624-2663
www.bones.nih.gov

**The North American Menopause
Society**
5900 Landerbrook Drive, Suite 390
Mayfield Heights, OH 44124
440-442-7550
www.menopause.org

North American Spine Society
7075 Veterans Blvd.
Burr Ridge, IL 60527
866-960-6277
www.spine.org

Womenshealth.gov
Office on Women's Health
U.S. Department of Health and Human
Services
200 Independence Ave., SW, Room 712E
Washington, DC 20201
800-994-9662
www.womenshealth.gov

Glossary

B

bisphosphonates. A family of drugs used to prevent and treat osteoporosis.

bone. An organ composed of living tissue comprised mostly of collagen and calcium; it provides structural support to the body.

bone density. The amount of calcium and minerals at a given site in the skeleton, divided by the area of bone at that site and measured in grams per square centimeter.

bone mass. The total amount of calcium and minerals in the skeleton.

bone mineral density test. Also called bone densitometry; it measures bone density to see if a person has low bone density or osteoporosis.

C

calcitonin. A hormone produced by the thyroid gland; it's also available as a medication to treat osteoporosis.

calcium. A mineral found in many foods that's used by the body to strengthen bone and teeth.

cancellous bone. Also called trabecular bone; this is the inner spongy part of bone that resembles a honeycomb.

collagen. An insoluble protein fiber that's the primary component in bone and connective tissues, such as skin and tendons.

compression fracture. A type of injury to the spine in which one or more vertebrae collapse.

cortical bone. The outer, hard layer of bone that surrounds the inner cancellous, or trabecular, bone.

D

dual energy X-ray absorptiometry (DXA). The most common technique used to measure bone mineral density.

E

elemental calcium. The amount of usable calcium contained in a calcium supplement.

endocrine system. The body system composed of glands that secrete hormones into blood.

estrogen. The major female sex hormone responsible for reproduction and development of secondary female sex characteristics.

F

femoral neck. The part of the hip-bone that connects the ball of the hip to the long shaft of the thighbone (femur).
fragility fractures. Fractures to bones that occur with minimal or no trauma.

G

glucocorticoid. A type of steroid medication used to treat asthma, rheumatoid arthritis and many other inflammatory diseases that can damage bone.

H

hyperparathyroidism. Excessive activity of the parathyroid glands.
hyperthyroidism. Excessive activity of the thyroid glands.
hypogonadism. Decreased activity of the male or female sex organs resulting in decreased testosterone or estrogen production.

K

kyphosis. Commonly called kyphotic curve or "humpback," the curve is a telltale sign of advanced osteoporosis caused by collapse of vertebrae.

M

menopause. The time in a woman's life when the ovaries shut down and stop producing the female hormones estrogen and progesterone.

O

ossification. The natural process of bone formation.
osteoblast. The type of cell that forms bone.
osteoclast. The type of cell that breaks down bone.
osteopenia. A condition in which there's a decrease in bone density but not to the point of osteoporosis.
osteoporosis. A condition in which there's a significant decrease in bone mass and bone density and an increased risk of bone fracture due to weakness in the bone.

P

parathyroid hormone. A hormone secreted by the parathyroid glands that increases blood calcium and may cause bone loss.
peak bone mass. The maximum amount of bone mass a person achieves during skeletal growth and development.

phosphorus. A mineral found in bone and many tissues that's also present in many foods.

postmenopausal. After menopause; this describes a woman whose periods have ended, whose ovaries have stopped producing eggs and whose hormone levels have decreased.

R

remodeling. The process of replacing old bone with new bone through the action of osteoclasts and osteoblasts.

resistance exercises. Exercises in which the muscle is acting against some form of resistance, as in lifting weights.

resorption. The breakdown and absorption of bone through the action of osteoclasts.

risk factors. Factors that influence an individual's risk of developing a condition or disease.

S

secondary osteoporosis. Bone loss caused by medications or other diseases or conditions; it's not related to normal aging.

spinal column. Also called the vertebral column; it extends from the skull to the pelvis and is made up of 33 individual bones called vertebrae.

standard deviation. A consistent unit of measure above or below the average of a comparison group.

T

testosterone. The major male sex hormone.

T-score. A measure of how far above or below a person's bone density is compared with young, healthy individuals of the same sex and ethnicity; measured in standard deviations.

V

vertebra. Any one of the 33 bony segments of the spinal column.

W

weight-bearing exercises. Exercises in which a person supports his or her own body weight.

Z

Z-score. A measure of how far above or below a person's bone density is compared with individuals of the same age, sex and ethnicity; measured in standard deviations.

Index

A

action plan
  benefits of, 97
  defined, 97
  developing, 97–110
  diet and nutrition, 98–107
  elements of, 97–98
  health behaviors, 110
  medications, 108–110
  objectives, 98
  physical activity, 107–108
  success, 98
age-related osteoporosis
  defined, 17
  degree of change, 20
  occurrence of, 20
aging
  balance and, 42–44
  bones and, 29–34
  chronic medical conditions and, 45–46
  falls and, 42
  muscle weakness and, 45
  as osteoporosis risk factor, 51, 90
  vision problems and, 44
alcohol use
  limiting, 34, 110, 130
  as osteoporosis risk factor, 61–62, 93
alendronate (Fosamax), 155
amenorrhea, 57, 178
anorexia nervosa, 60
antibody to sclerostin, 162
anticonvulsants, 54–55
anxiety, 196
appearance, 199
aromatase inhibitors, 56
artificial hip joints, 213
assistive devices
  in bathroom, 229
  canes, 230–231
  for daily needs, 228–229
  finding, 227–228
  function of, 227
  grips and tips, 232
  for movement and mobility, 229
  open mind and, 232–233
  taking time and, 232
  walkers, 231–232
  See also home safety
attitude, in home safety, 233–234

B

back-strengthening exercises, 144
balance
  falls and, 42–44
  reaction to medications and, 46
  sensory systems, 42
bed rest
  prolonged, 58
  in vertebral fracture recovery, 209
biceps curls, 143
biofeedback, 221
bisphosphonates
  defined, 151, 239
  fractures and, 154
  how long should you take? 155
  ibandronate, 151
  infusion, 151–153
  for men with osteoporosis, 174
  oral, 151
  risks of long-term use, 153
  safety, 154
  taking, 152
  type selection, 153
  zoledronic acid, 151
  See also medications
blood clots, hip fractures and, 39
blood thinners, 55
body size, as osteoporosis risk factor, 53, 92
bone
  aging and, 29–34
  brittleness, 32
  builders, 23
  building with physical activity, 107–108
  cortical, 22, 23, 239
  defined, 239
  life stages and, 21
  membrane, 22
  outside surface, 22
  structure, 22
  tissue, 22
  trabecular, 22, 23–24
bone anti-resorptive agents, 108
bone bank
  defined, 14
  not enough bone in, 14–15
  transactions, 14
  withdrawals, 15
bone biopsies, 73

bone breakdown, 24, 26
bone cycle
    aging and, 29–34
    bone remodeling and, 24–26
    hormones and, 26–28
    influencing, 34
    overview of, 21
    peak bone density, 28–29, 34
bone densitometers
    dual energy X-ray absorptiometry (DXA),
        70–71, 72
    high-resolution magnetic resonance imaging
        (micro-MRI), 75
    high-resolution pQCT (HRpQCT), 75
    peripheral, 73–75
    peripheral dual energy X-ray absorptiometry
        (pDXA), 74
    peripheral quantitative computerized tomography
        (pQCT), 74
    quantitative computerized tomography (QCT),
        71–73
    quantitative ultrasound (QUS), 74
    types of, 70–75
bone density
    defined, 14, 239
    low, 20, 47
    in men, 165–167
    mineral content and, 65
    peak, 28–29
    rise and fall of, 30
bone density tests
    annual, 67
    defined, 65, 81, 239
    determination of right one, 76–77
    diagnosis and, 94
    frequency of, 66
    government assistance for, 69
    how to get tested, 67–68
    location for, 67–68
    in men, 170
    at menopause, 66
    mineral content snapshot, 67
    osteoporosis and, 77
    payment for, 68
    process of, 68–70
    recommendations, 66
    risk factors and, 76
    sites for, 65
    time for, 70
    who should be tested, 65–67
    X-rays and, 69
    See also test results
bone formation
    bone breakdown and, 26
    in bone remodeling cycle, 24–25
    hormones and, 26–28

    illustrated, 26
    PTH (parathyroid hormone) in, 27–28
bone healing
    illustrated, 207
    phases of, 206–207
bone health
    factors, 49–50
    nutrients and, 113
bone loss
    age-related, 17–20
    defined, 15
    equilibrium shift to, 28
    in men, 167
    menopause and, 33
    osteoporosis and, 15
    reasons for, 17
    transition from bone gain to, 30
bone marker tests
    candidates for, 79
    defined, 78
    formation markers, 80
    how it works, 78–79
    resorption markers, 79–80
    serum bone specific alkaline phosphatase and
        serum osteocalcin, 80
    serum CTx-telopeptide (CTx), 79
    serum or urine NTx-telopeptide (NTx), 80
    serum procollagen carboxy terminal extension
        peptide (P1NP), 80
    types of, 79–80
bone marrow, 24
bone mass
    building while young, 29
    building with physical activity, 131
    defined, 14, 239
    loss of, 17
    low, 20
    peak, 17
    young adult men versus women, 51
bone quality, fracture risk and, 45
bone remodeling
    cycle, 25
    defined, 24, 241
    genes and, 34
    hormones in, 26–28
    reasons for occurrence of, 24
    stages, 24–25
bone scans, 73
bone strength
    defined, 14
    maintenance of, 28
bone-healthy meals, 118–119
bracing, in vertebral fracture recovery,
        209
breakfast, in bone-healthy meals, 118, 119
broken bones. See fractures

C

caffeine, 130
calcitonin, 160, 239
calcium
    absorption, 103
    in bone health, 23
    cheese, 116
    as cornerstone in treatment, 109
    dairy products, 114, 116
    deficiency, reasons for, 101
    defined, 239
    elemental, 239
    fish and shellfish, 116
    foods adding, 115
    fruits, 116
    how much are you getting? 115
    increasing in diet, 102
    increasing intake, 124–125
    loss of, 100
    low, signs and symptoms, 158
    for men with osteoporosis, 173
    overview of, 100
    pregnancy and lactation and, 102
    prostate cancer and, 128
    recommended daily, 101
    requirements, 100–101
    sources of, 114–117
    vegetables, 117
    See also diet and nutrition
calcium supplements
    absorbability, 127
    amount of calcium, 126–127
    choosing, 126–129
    combined with vitamins, 126
    examples of, 128
    form of, 127
    heart disease and, 128
    not overdoing, 102, 129
    quality and cost, 127
    recommendation, 125
    risks of, 127–129
    tolerability, 127
    types of, 125–126
cancellous bone, 239
cancer, 181–184
canes
    grips and tips, 232
    height, 230
    using, 230–231
casts, 217
cathepsin K inhibitors, 162
central densitometers
    dual energy X-ray absorptiometry (DXA), 70–71, 72
    quantitative computerized tomography (QCT), 71–73
    See also bone densitometers

chair situps, 143
childbearing, as osteoporosis risk factor, 54
children, fractures in, 41
chiropractic treatments, 109
chronic medical conditions
    falls and, 45–46
    osteoporosis in men and, 168
chronic obstructive pulmonary disease (COPD), 168
chronic pain management
    alternative methods for, 220–222
    biofeedback in, 221
    challenges of, 219
    electrical stimulation in, 222
    exercise in, 221
    ice and heat in, 221
    medications and, 220
    music therapy in, 221–222
    pain disappearance and, 219
    relaxation techniques in, 221
    your role in, 219
collagen, 239
Colles' fracture
    defined, 40, 215
    recovery from, 41
    signs and symptoms of, 41
complementary and alternative treatments, 109
compression fractures
    defined, 239
    illustrated, 16, 37
    multiple, signs of, 37
    occurrence of, 37
    osteoporosis and, 16, 37
    signs and symptoms, 16
    undetected, 37
COPD (chronic obstructive pulmonary disease), 168
coping strategies
    anger management, 200–202
    education, 200
    exercise, 200
    positive thinking, 200
    relaxation, 200
    types of, 198–202
cortical bone, 22, 23, 239
corticosteroids, 54–55
coughing, 192
Cushing's syndrome, 56, 178

D

daily tasks
    assistive devices for, 228–229
    safety tips for, 195
denosumab (Prolia)
    defined, 154, 157
    delivery, 154
    side effects, 158
    taking, 158

use of, 157–158
See also medications
densitometers. *See* bone densitometers
depression, 196–198
diagnosis
  bone density tests and, 94
  making, 80
diagnostic tests
  bone density, 64, 65–70
  bone marker, 78–80
  defined, 64
  results from, 64
  screening tests versus, 64
diet and nutrition
  in action plan, 98–107
  alcohol and, 130
  bone health and, 113
  bone-healthy meals, 118–119
  caffeine and, 130
  calcium, 100–102, 114–117
  fat, 112–114
  foods to avoid, 129–130
  in fracture recovery, 215
  fruits, 112
  good, 111–115
  for healthy bones, 111–130
  in peak bone density, 29, 34
  phosphorus, 106, 129–130
  protein, 106–107, 112–114
  recipes, 120–121
  salt, 129
  sodium, 106
  starting young and, 99
  sugar, 129
  vegetables, 112
  vitamin D, 103–105
  whole grains, 112
dieting, as osteoporosis risk factor, 60
disorders associated with osteoporosis
  cancer, 181–184
  drugs and, 182–183
  endocrine disorders, 177–178
  gastrointestinal disorders, 178
  genetic diseases, 184
  glucocorticoid-related disease, 179–180
  immobility, 186
  kidney disorders, 181
  kyphosis, 184–186
  liver disorders, 180
  overview of, 177
  rheumatologic disorders, 179
  transplant surgery, 181
diuretics, 55
doctor consultations, 133
dual energy X-ray absorptiometry (DXA)
  accuracy, 71, 76

  defined, 70, 239
  of hip, 80, 85
  illustrated, 72
  location for, 71
  for men, 170
  process of, 70–71
  of spine, 76, 82

E
eating disorders, as osteoporosis risk factor, 58–61
education, 200
electrical stimulation, 222
emotional health
  anger, 198
  appearance and, 199
  coping strategies, 198–202
  depression, 196–198
  fear and anxiety, 196
  self-esteem, 198
  stress and, 197
  See also healthy living strategies
endocrine disorders, 56, 177–178, 182
endocrine system, 239
endocrinologists, 68
environmental hazards, 46
estrogen
  declining levels of, 33
  defined, 239
  factor, 33–34
  role, 33
exercise buddies, 148
exercise(s)
  amount of, 145–147
  back-strengthening, 144
  choosing, 147
  in chronic pain management, 221
  classes, 147
  cooling down, 138
  as coping strategy, 200
  danger signs during, 135
  defined, 132
  doctor consultation and, 133
  duration of, 147
  fitness assessment before, 134
  frequency of, 145
  getting started with, 133–137
  goals, 134–135
  importance of, 131–132
  intensity of, 145
  isometric, 141
  lapses, 148
  listening to body and, 137
  for men with osteoporosis, 172, 173–174
  milestones, 148
  motivation, 147–148
  for osteoporosis, 138–145

exercise(s) continued
>   pacing, 137
>   resistance, 140–145
>   risk movements, avoiding, 135–136
>   scheduling, 137
>   six-month plan, 147
>   starting slowly, 136
>   stretching, 146
>   variety to routine, 147
>   in vertebral fracture recovery, 209–210
>   walking, 139
>   warming up, 138
>   weight-bearing, 138–139
>   *See also* physical activity
external fixation, 217

F

falls
>   aging and, 42
>   balance problems and, 42–44
>   in breaking bones, 42
>   chronic medical conditions and, 45–46
>   environmental hazards and, 46
>   hip fractures and, 43
>   muscle weakness and, 45
>   poor bone quality and, 45
>   reaction to medications and, 46
>   steps for preventing, 225
>   vision problems and, 44
family history, as osteoporosis risk factor, 92
fat, 112–114
fear, 196
femoral neck fractures, 211, 240
fitness assessment, 134
flexibility, 146
formation markers, 80
forward bending, 135–136
fracture recovery
>   activity, 215
>   bone healing process, 206–207
>   chronic pain management and, 219
>   diet and, 215
>   general concerns, 212–213
>   hip fractures, 211–215
>   at home, 214–215
>   at the hospital, 213–214
>   incision cleanliness, 214
>   overview of, 205
>   process of, 205–206
>   prosthesis in, 213, 214–215
>   swelling and, 214
>   vertebral fractures, 208–211
>   wrist fractures, 215–222
fractures, 36–41
>   avoiding, 46–47
>   bone quality and, 45

Colles', 40–41
>   common sites, 36, 65
>   compression, 16, 36–39
>   as first indication of osteoporosis, 12
>   fragility, 240
>   hip, 36, 39–40, 211–215
>   kids and, 41
>   as life changing, 48
>   low-trauma, 48
>   mechanisms of, 43
>   occurrence of, 35, 36
>   as osteoporosis indication, 35
>   preventing, 48
>   previous, 92
>   risk determination, 91, 93
>   spinal, 36–39
>   treatment, 216
>   vertebral, 208–211
>   wrist, 36, 40–41, 215–222
fragility fractures, 240
FRAX, 91
free weights, 140–141
fruits, 112

G

gastrointestinal disorders, 57, 178, 182
genetic diseases, 182–183, 184
genetics, osteoporosis in men and, 169
glucocorticoids, 240
glucocorticoids use, 93
glucocorticoid-related disease, 179–180
goals, exercise, 134–135
gonadotrophin-releasing hormone agonists, 56
growth factors, 163
growth hormone (somatotropin), 162

H

hazards, environmental, 46
healthy behaviors, 108–110
healthy living strategies
>   emotional health, 196–202
>   good posture, 189–191
>   safe movement, 191
>   social connections, 201, 202–204
heavy lifting, 136
heredity
>   as osteoporosis risk factor, 52–53
>   in peak bone density, 29
high-impact activities, 136
high-resolution magnetic resonance imaging
>   (micro-MRI), 75
high-resolution pQCT (HRpQCT), 75
hip fractures
>   blood clots and, 39
>   complications from, 39

falling sideways and, 43
from falls, 36
family history of, 92
femoral neck, 211
illustrated, 40
internal fixation, 211
intertrochanteric region, 211–212
locations, 39
in men, 19
partial hip replacement, 211
prosthesis, 213
recovery from, 39–40, 211–215
total hip replacement, 211
treatment options for, 212
white postmenopausal women and, 53
X-ray confirmation, 39
See also fractures
hip joints, artificial, 213
hip surgery
general concerns, 213
at home, 214–215
at the hospital, 213–214
home safety
assistive devices, 227–233
attitude, 233–234
clear pathways, 224
fall prevention, 225
importance of, 223
lighting, 224–226
seating, 226
survey, 224
taking control of, 234
work areas, 226–227
hormone replacement therapy, 150
hormone-related therapy, 150
hormones
bone formation and, 26–28
defined, 26–27
as osteoporosis risk factor, 53
production, in peak bone density, 29
HRpQCT (high resolution pQCT), 75
hunchback. *See* kyphosis
hyperparathyroidism, 56, 178, 240
hyperthyroidism, 178, 240
hypogonadism, 56, 178, 240

I
ibandronate (Boniva), 151
ice and heat, 221
immobilization, 183, 186
inflammatory disorders, 178
injectable bone cement, 217–218
internal fixation, 211, 217
intertrochanteric region fractures, 211–212
intestinal disorders, 57
isometric exercise, 141

K
kidney disorders, 181, 182
kyphoplasty, 210–211
kyphosis
curve severity, 186
defined, 177, 184, 240
risk of, 184–185
treatment for, 185

L
lactose intolerance, 30–32, 57, 126
lifestyle
bone-saving changes, 34
osteoporosis in men and, 168–169
in peak bone density, 29
lifting, 192–193
lighting, in home safety, 224–226
liver disorders, 57, 180, 182
long-handled objects, 194
lower back extensions, 144
low-impact weight-bearing activities, 137
low-trauma fractures, 48

M
magnesium, 23
malabsorption disorders, 178
massage, 109
meals, bone-healthy, 118–119
medical conditions
amenorrhea, 57
chronic, 45–46
Cushing's syndrome, 56, 178
endocrine disorders, 56, 177–178, 182
gastrointestinal disorders, 57, 178, 182
hyperparathyroidism, 56, 178, 240
hypogonadism, 56, 178, 240
intestinal disorders, 57
lactose intolerance, 30–32, 57, 126
liver disorders, 57, 180, 182
osteoporosis and, 18
as osteoporosis risk factor, 56–57
in peak bone density, 29
rheumatoid arthritis, 57, 93
type 1 diabetes, 56, 178
medical history, 77
medications
in action plan, 108–110
antibody to sclerostin, 162
anticonvulsants, 54–55
aromatase inhibitors, 56
bisphosphonates, 151–154, 155
blood thinners, 55
bone anti-resorptive agents, 108
bone density tests and, 77
calcitonin, 160
cathepsin K, 162

medications continued
   in chronic pain management, 220
   corticosteroids, 54–55
   denosumab, 157–158
   disorders associated with osteoporosis and, 182–183
   diuretics, 55
   getting the most from, 161–164
   glucocorticoids, 179–180
   gonadotrophin-releasing hormone agonists, 56
   growth hormones and growth factors, 162–163
   under investigation, 162–163
   osteoporosis and, 18, 149
   osteoporosis in men and, 167–168
   as osteoporosis risk factor, 54–56
   raloxifene, 158–159
   reaction to, 46
   taking, 149–164
   teriparatide, 154–157
   thiazide diuretics, 161
   thyroid medicine, 55
   vitamin D analogues, 162
men
   estrogen levels and, 33
   hormones as risk factor, 53
   peak bone mass, 33–34
   screening in, 169–171
   See also osteoporosis in men
menopause
   bone density tests at, 66
   bone loss after, 33
   defined, 240
   going through, 33
   smokers and, 61
micro-MRI (high-resolution magnetic resonance imaging), 75
milk
   as calcium source, 114, 116
   in cooking, 125
   myths, 122
minerals
   content, 65
   defined, 23
   importance of, 23
motivation, exercise, 147–148
movement and mobility devices, 229
moving meditation, 109
moving safely
   coughing and sneezing, 192
   long-handled objects and, 194
   overview of, 191–192
   pushing and pulling, 194
   sleeping, 192–193
   working and lifting, 192–193
muscle weakness, 45
music therapy, 221–222

O

obesity, as osteoporosis risk factor, 58
oral bisphosphonates, 151
organ transplants, 57–58
ossification, 240
osteoarthritis, 15
osteoblasts
   in bone remodeling cycle, 26
   defined, 25, 240
osteoclasts
   in bone remodeling cycle, 26
   defined, 25, 240
   illustrated, 26
osteopenia, 240
osteoporosis
   age-related, 17–20
   body weight and, 105
   bone loss and, 15, 17
   changes with age and, 12
   compression fractures and, 16
   defined, 11, 240
   disorders associated with, 177–186
   exercises for, 138–145
   in history, 13
   hormone replacement therapy and, 150
   osteoarthritis versus, 15
   overview of, 11
   postmenopausal, 17
   prevalence of, 12
   risk evaluation for, 59
   risks, 12
   secondary, 18, 20, 241
   signs and symptoms, 15–16
   as silent thief, 15
   statistics, 11
   successful avoidance of, 11
   types of, 17–20
osteoporosis in men
   bisphosphonates and, 174
   bone density and, 165–166
   calcium and, 173
   chronic illness and, 168
   digestive disorders and, 168
   disability and mortality rate, 165
   evaluation, 170
   exercise and, 172, 173–174
   genetics and, 169
   hormone disorders and, 168
   increasing numbers of, 165
   lack of menopause and, 166
   lifestyle habits and, 168–169
   medications and, 167–168
   occurrence of, 167–169
   peak bone mass, 166
   quality of bone loss, 167
   screening, 169–171

self-care, 175
signs and symptoms of, 169
statistics, 19
taking action and, 176
teriparatide and, 175
test results, 170–171
testosterone replacement and, 175
treatment, 171–175
vitamin D and, 173

P

pain relievers, in vertebral fracture recovery, 208
parathyroid glands, 28
parathyroid hormone (PTH), 27–28, 154–156, 240
partial hip replacement, 211
pathways, clear, 224
pDXA (peripheral dual energy X-ray absorptiometry), 74
peak bone density
  defined, 28
  influences, 29
  maximizing, 34
  in men, 166
  osteoporosis protection and, 29
peak bone mass
  defined, 240
  factors that reduce, 50
pelvic tilts, 144
periosteum, 22
peripheral densitometers
  high-resolution magnetic resonance imaging (micro-MRI), 75
  high-resolution pQCT (HRpQCT), 75
  peripheral dual energy X-ray absorptiometry (pDXA), 74
  peripheral quantitative computerized tomography (pQCT), 74
  quantitative ultrasound (QUS), 74
  See also bone densitometers
peripheral dual energy X-ray absorptiometry (pDXA), 74
peripheral quantitative computerized tomography (pQCT), 74
phosphate, 23
phosphorus, 106, 129–130, 241
physical activity
  in action plan, 107–108
  in building bone, 107–108, 131
  defined, 132
  high-impact, 136
  importance of, 131–132
  lack of as osteoporosis risk factor, 61
  low-impact weight-bearing, 137
  in maximizing peak bone density, 34
  as part of family routine, 99
  in peak bone density, 29

posture and, 108
routine tasks as, 132
structured, 108
See also exercise(s)
physical exam, 77
physical therapy, wrist fractures and, 218
positive outlook, 20
positive thinking, 200
postmenopausal, 241
postmenopausal osteoporosis, 17
posture
  defined, 108
  good, practicing, 189–191
  perfecting, 108
  sitting, 190
  standing, 190, 191
  tips for improving, 191–192
pQCT (peripheral quantitative computerized tomography), 74
pregnancy
  alcohol and, 130
  calcium and, 102
previous fracture, as osteoporosis risk factor, 92
prolonged bed rest, 58
protein
  as bone building block, 106–107
  limiting, 112–114
  overconsumption of, 106–107
PTH (parathyroid hormone), 27–28, 240
pushing and pulling, 194

Q

quantitative computerized tomography (QCT), 71–73
quantitative ultrasound (QUS), 74

R

race
  as osteoporosis risk factor, 53
  in peak bone density, 29
raloxifene (Evista)
  defined, 158
  SERMs and, 158–159
  side effects, 159
  taking, 159
  use of, 159
reacher, 228
reaching overhead, 136
recipes
  chocolate ricotta mousse, 120
  spinach with feta cheese and almonds, 121
  tropical smoothie, 121
  wild rice soup, 120
relaxation
  in chronic pain management, 221
  as coping strategy, 200

remodeling. *See* bone remodeling
resistance bands, 141
resistance exercises
    bands, 141
    biceps curls, 143
    chair situps, 143
    defined, 140, 241
    importance of, 142
    isometric exercise, 141
    need for, 140
    performing, 142
    training program, 140
    wall pushups, 143
    water, 142
    weight training, 140–141
    whole-body vibration, 142–145
    See also exercise(s)
resorption, 241
resorption markers
    defined, 79
    serum CTx-telopeptide (CTx), 79
    serum or urine NTx-telopeptide (NTx), 80
    See also bone marker tests
resources, 235–238
rheumatoid arthritis, 57, 93
rheumatologic disorders, 179, 182
risk
    evaluation for osteoporosis, 59
    fracture, 91
    reducing, 49–62
    understanding, 50
risk factors
    age, 90
    alcohol use, 61–62, 93
    body frame, 92
    bone density tests and, 76
    changeable, 58–62
    childbearing, 54
    defined, 50, 241
    eating disorders, 58–61
    family history, 92
    glucocorticoid use, 93
    influenceable, 54–58
    medical conditions, 56–57
    medications, 54–56
    obesity, 58
    physical activity, 61
    previous fracture, 92
    prolonged bed rest, 58
    rheumatoid arthritis, 93
    sex, 50–51, 90–92
    smoking, 61, 93
    surgical procedures, 57–58
    unchangeable, 50–53
    weight and dieting, 58–61
risky movements, avoiding, 135–136

S
safety
    assistive devices, 227–233
    coughing and sneezing, 192
    for daily tasks, 195
    home, 223–234
    long-handled objects and, 194
    moving, 191–195
    pushing and pulling, 194
    sleeping, 192–193
    working and lifting, 192–193
salt, 129
sclerostin, 162
screening tests, 64
seating, safe, 226
secondary causes
    medical conditions and, 18
    medications and, 18
    reasons for, 20
    statistics, 20
    surgical procedures and, 18
secondary osteoporosis, 93, 241
selective estrogen receptor modulators (SERMs), 158–159
self-care, men with osteoporosis, 175
self-esteem, 198
serum bone specific alkaline phosphatase and serum osteocalcin, 80
serum CTx-telopeptide (CTx), 79
serum or urine NTx-telopeptide (NTx), 80
serum procollagen carboxy terminal extension peptide (P1NP), 80
sex
    as osteoporosis risk factor, 50–51, 90–92
    in peak bone density, 29
shrinking, 31
sitting posture, 190
sleeping, 192–193
smoking
    avoiding, 110
    as osteoporosis risk factor, 61, 93
    as osteoporosis risk factor in men, 168–169
snacks, in bone-healthy meals, 118, 119
sneezing, 192
social connections
    bolstering, 201
    maintaining, 202–204
    osteoporosis consequences, 202–203
    reaching out, 203
    support group, 203–204
sodium, 106
soft drinks, 129
soy isoflavones, 109
spinal column, 241
spinal fractures, 36–39
spine, 38

splints, 217
standard deviations, 85, 87, 241
standing posture, 190, 191
steroids, 180
stress management, 197
stretching exercises, 146
sugar, 129
support groups, 203–204
surgical procedures
    gastric surgery, 58
    organ transplants, 57–58
    as osteoporosis risk factor, 57–58
    as secondary osteoporosis cause, 18

T

tai chi, 109
TENS (transcutaneous electrical nerve stimulation), 222
teriparatide (Forteo)
    as anabolic agent, 156
    defined, 154
    expense of, 157
    for men with osteoporosis, 175
    optimal length of treatment, 156–157
    PTH and, 154–156
    side effects, 156
    taking, 156
    See also medications
test results
    black square on graph, 83, 85
    colored graph, 82–83
    DXA images, 82, 84
    elements of, 81–82
    in fracture risk, 91
    FRAX and, 91
    images, 82
    in men, 170–171
    number examples, 88–90
    revealing osteoporosis, 84
    summary table, 82
    T-scores, 85–87
    white lines, 83, 84
    Z-scores, 87–88
    See also bone density tests
testosterone, 241
testosterone replacement, 175
thiazide diuretics, 161
thyroid medicine, 55
total hip replacement, 211
trabecular bone, 22, 23–24
transcutaneous electrical nerve stimulation (TENS), 222
transplant surgery, 181
T-scores
    defined, 85, 241
    from different bones, 86

    interpreting, 87
    in low bone density evaluation, 86
    in men, 170–171
    normal Z-scores and, 88
    number usage, 88–90
    numbers, 86
    standard deviations, 85
    understanding, 85–87
    See also test results
twisting, 136
type 1 diabetes, 56, 178

U

upper back extensions, 144

V

vegetables, 112
vertebrae, 38, 241
vertebral fractures
    bed rest and, 209
    bracing and, 209
    exercise and, 209–210
    kyphoplasty, 210–211
    occurrence of, 36–39
    pain relievers and, 208
    recovery from, 208–211
    vertebroplasty, 210
    See also fractures
vertebroplasty, 210
vision problems, 44
vitamin D
    body production of, 32, 103
    as cornerstone in treatment, 109
    deficiency, 104–105
    importance of, 103
    for men with osteoporosis, 173
    recommended daily, 104
    requirements, 104–105
    sources of, 103–104
    from sunlight, 103, 105
    See also diet and nutrition
vitamin D analogues, 162

W

walkers
    alignment, 231–232
    defined, 231
    grips and tips, 232
    walking with, 232
    with wheels, 231
walking, 139
wall pushups, 143
water workouts, 142
weight
    osteoporosis and, 105
    as osteoporosis risk factor, 58

weight training, 140–141
weight-bearing activities, 186
weight-bearing exercises
    aerobic benefits, 139
    defined, 138, 241
    impact precaution, 138
    walking, 139
    See also exercise(s)
whole-body vibration, 142–145
whole grains, 112
women
    hormones as risk factor, 53
    peak bone mass, 33
    postmenopausal osteoporosis, 17
work areas, organizing, 226–227
wrist fractures
    cast or splint, 217
    Colles', 40–41
    complexity, 215–217
    complications from, 41
    external fixation, 217
    from falls, 36
    illustrated, 41, 218
    injectable bone cement, 217–218
    internal fixation, 217
    location of, 40
    physical therapy, 218
    recovery from, 41, 215–222
    signs and symptoms of, 41
    See also fractures

X

X-rays
    bone density tests and, 69
    bones of different densities, 71

Z

zoledronic acid (Reclast, Zometa), 151
Z-scores
    abnormal T-scores and, 88
    defined, 85, 241
    indications from, 87
    in men, 171
    number usage, 88–90
    numbers, 87–88
    standard deviations, 87
    See also test results

MAYO CLINIC

Housecall

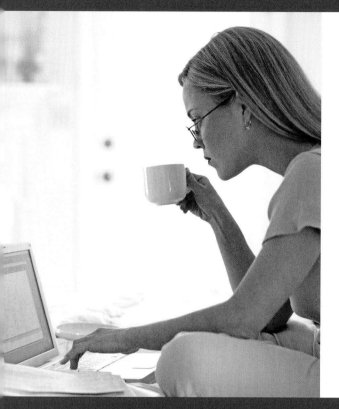

What our readers are saying ...

*"I depend on **Mayo Clinic Housecall** more than any other medical info that shows up on my computer. Thank you so very much."*

"Excellent newsletter. I always find something interesting to read and learn something new."

*"**Housecall** is a must read – keep up the good work!"*

*"I love **Housecall**. It is one of the most useful, trusted and beneficial things that come from the Internet."*

*"The **Housecall** is timely, interesting and invaluable in its information. Thanks much to Mayo Clinic for this resource!"*

"I enjoy getting the weekly newsletters. They provide me with friendly reminders, as well as information/ conditions I was not aware of."

Get the latest health information direct from Mayo Clinic ... Sign up today, it's FREE!

Mayo Clinic Housecall is a FREE weekly e-newsletter that offers the latest health information from the experts at Mayo Clinic. Stay up to date on topics that are current, interesting, and most of all important to your health and the health of your family.

What you get
- Weekly top story
- Additional healthy highlights
- Answers from the experts
- Quick access to trusted health tools
- Featured blogs
- Health tip of the week
- Special offers

Don't wait ... Join today!
MayoClinic.com/Housecall/Register

We're committed to helping you enjoy better health and get the most out of life every day. We hope you decide to become part of the Mayo Clinic family, where you can always count on receiving an interesting mix of health information from a trusted source.

More great Mayo Clinic publications

Visit **www.store.MayoClinic.com** for reliable Mayo Clinic publications to help with your top health interests.

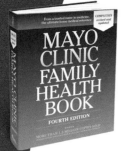

Mayo Clinic Family Health Book
Completely revised and updated Fourth Edition
It's your owner's manual for the human body.

Mayo Clinic Healthy Heart for Life
Start improving your heart health in as little as 10 minutes a day.

The Mayo Clinic Diet
#1 New York Times Best Seller
The last diet you'll ever need!

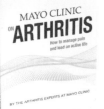

Mayo Clinic on Arthritis
Better medications, improved treatments and self-care tips to lead a more active, comfortable life.

Many more popular titles to choose from ...

» Mayo Clinic on Healthy Aging

» Mayo Clinic on Alzheimer's Disease

» The Mayo Clinic Breast Cancer Book

» Mayo Clinic Essential Diabetes Book

» The Mayo Clinic Diabetes Diet

» The Mayo Clinic Diabetes Diet Journal

» Mayo Clinic on Digestive Health

» Mayo Clinic Fitness for EveryBody

» Fix-It And Enjoy-It Healthy Cookbook

» Mayo Clinic Guide to Your Baby's First Year

» Mayo Clinic Guide to a Healthy Pregnancy

» Mayo Clinic on Better Hearing and Balance

» Mayo Clinic 5 Steps to Controlling High Blood Pressure

» Mayo Clinic Book of Home Remedies

» Mayo Clinic on Managing Incontinence

» The Mayo Clinic Kids' Cookbook

» The New Mayo Clinic Cookbook

» The Mayo Clinic Diet Journal

» Mayo Clinic Guide to Preventing and Treating Osteoporosis

» Mayo Clinic Essential Guide to Prostate Health

» Mayo Clinic Guide to Better Vision

Learn more at
www.store.MayoClinic.com